AMBULATORY SURGERY

Developing and Managing Successful Programs

Contributors

Marlene J. Berkoff, AIA
Eric N. Berkowitz, Ph.D.
Linda A. Burns, M.H.A.
Sharon M. Buske, R.N., B.S.N.
James E. Davis, M.D.
Mindy S. Ferber, M.B.A.
Douglas D. Hawthorne, M.S.

James O. Jonassen, AIA
M. Robert Knapp, M.D., F.A.C.P.
Richard O. Kraft, M.D., F.A.C.S.
James W. Maher
Eleanor Nealon
Mark V. Pauly, Ph.D.
Steven Sieverts

AMBULATORY SURGERY

Developing and Managing Successful Programs

Linda A. Burns

Director
Division of Ambulatory Care
American Hospital Association

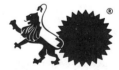

AN ASPEN PUBLICATION®

Aspen Systems Corporation
Rockville, Maryland
Royal Tunbridge Wells
1984

Library of Congress Cataloging in Publication Data

Burns, Linda A.
Ambulatory surgery.

Includes indexes.
1. Surgery, Outpatient.   2. Hospitals—United States—
Outpatient services—Administration.   I. Title
[DNLM: 1. Ambulatory surgery.   2. Organization
and Administration. WO 192 A4975]
RD110.B87 1984   362.1'97   83-19732
ISBN: 0-89443-897-2

Publisher: John Marozsan
Editor-in-Chief: Michael Brown
Executive Managing Editor: Margot Raphael
Editorial Services: Jane Coyle
Printing and Manufacturing: Debbie Collins

Library of Congress Catalog Card Number: 83-19732
ISBN: 0-89443-897-2

Printed in the United States of America

1 2 3 4 5

Table of Contents

Preface

Ambulatory surgery programs, sponsored by hospitals or by providers organized independently of hospitals, can be found in all regions of the country in growing numbers. The question now facing hospitals and other providers is not whether to offer such a program, but rather how the program should be developed and managed in order to be most successful. Factors to be considered in the development of ambulatory surgery centers include financial viability and price competitiveness, convenience and satisfaction of patients, suitability for physicians, assurance of quality of care, and compliance with regulatory and voluntary accreditation standards.

This book addresses important factors to consider in developing successful ambulatory surgery programs. It provides information on ambulatory surgery programs throughout the United States. It includes chapters on marketing, facility planning and design, the surgeon's role and perspective in planning and participating in an ambulatory surgery program, a review of consumers' perspectives, a discussion of a Blue Cross and Blue Shield Plan to pay for ambulatory surgery, and three case studies. The book concludes with a discussion of how financial incentives for hospitals, physicians, and patients might be constructed to encourage the substitution of ambulatory surgery for inpatient surgery.

In the future, ambulatory surgery programs can be expected to grow. Technological advances, incentives for efficiency through health financing mechanisms, and consumer preferences are expected to spur the growth of ambulatory surgery in the years ahead. The implementation of prospective pricing and the development of other financial incentive plans such as copayments and coinsurance will encourage both hospitals and physicians to develop ambulatory surgery programs and to operate them efficiently.

Linda A. Burns

Chapter 1

Ambulatory Surgery in the United States: Trends and Developments

Linda A. Burns, M.H.A.
Mindy S. Ferber, M.B.A.

The concept of ambulatory surgery is far from new. At a meeting of the British Medical Association in 1909, J. H. Nicoll, M.D., reviewed 7,320 operations that he had performed on ambulatory patients at the Royal Glasgow Hospital for Children. In 1980 there were over 19 million surgical procedures performed in community hospitals in the United States.[1] Not too many years ago, each of these procedures would have required an overnight stay in the hospital. As a result of significant technological advances and an era of cost consciousness, ambulatory surgery has gained wide acceptance and accounts for a significant portion of the number of surgical procedures performed in hospitals as well as in independent health facilities.

Within the past twenty years, several major developments have contributed to the acceptance of ambulatory surgery by the medical community, and have encouraged the proliferation of ambulatory surgery programs by hospitals and other providers. The pharmaceutical industry has developed anesthetics that act rapidly, leaving the patient with minimal prolonged side effects, such as drowsiness and transient, but occasionally profound, nausea. In addition, the availability and use of short-acting narcotic and nonnarcotic analgesics to treat pain and of drugs to manage nausea and vomiting have reduced patient discomfort. Moreover, surgeons have been encouraging patients to become ambulatory soon after surgery, resulting in decreased recovery time. Evidence also exists that good perioperative teaching by nurses and physicians has created a smoother postoperative recovery and reduced the length of inpatient stay.

Adapted from *Journal of Ambulatory Care Management* 1981, 3:1–13.

DEFINITIONS

Ambulatory surgery is defined here as scheduled surgical procedures provided to patients who do not remain in the hospital overnight. Although surgery not requiring an overnight hospital stay is often performed in private physicians' offices, hospital emergency departments, and free-standing, independent emergency centers, this chapter addresses *organized* ambulatory surgery programs—in other words, programs specifically designed and managed to provide scheduled surgical procedures to ambulatory patients.

Organized ambulatory surgery programs are offered by hospitals as well as by independent providers. Obviously, a program that is managed and governed for the primary purpose of providing ambulatory surgery is an *organized* program. In contrast to independent, freestanding ambulatory surgery centers or programs, organized ambulatory surgery programs in hospitals can take various forms.

An organized program in a hospital has, for example, one or more of the following characteristics: a separate cost center; a separate facility or specifically designated surgical suites; an independent patient registration system; independent preoperative and postoperative settings. Surgical procedures can be performed in a variety of facilities, including the inpatient operating room suites (ORs), separate ORs dedicated to ambulatory surgery, a freestanding facility, or the emergency department.

Degree of Control

When discussing hospital involvement in ambulatory surgery, it is necessary to specify the degree of control the individual hospital exercises over its ambulatory surgery program. A high degree of control is found in a hospital that has corporate ownership of the program, provides the management, and makes the major policy decisions. A low degree of control or involvement is apparent in a hospital that owns the facility in which the ambulatory surgery program resides and rents or leases the facility to medical professionals, who then operate and manage the ambulatory surgery program. Hospital-owned physician office buildings are an example of this type of involvement.

Of critical importance in determining the degree of hospital involvement is the extent to which the hospital controls physician services. A hospital that hires and salaries physicians to provide defined ambulatory services exercises a greater degree of control over the manner and quality of those services than a hospital that does not. A hospital that does not have physicians on its payroll, however, may still achieve a high degree of control over its ambulatory care program, to the extent that the hospital is able to place the individual physician or medical group providing services at financial risk or gain through contractual arrangements. In other words, the hospital may be able to fashion an agreement whereby the hospital and physicians share the financial losses and gains from a program's operation.

Basic Categories

Ambulatory surgery programs have been divided into the following categories, based on their governance, management, and source of financing:[2]

- *Hospital sponsored:* The program is completely governed, managed, and financed by the hospital.
- *Hospital associated:* The program is governed and managed by the hospital but financed through a contractual arrangement of shared expenses and revenues with physicians.
- *Hospital as landlord:* The physical facility in which the program is located is owned by the hospital, but the ambulatory services are not governed, managed, or financed by the hospital.

Another set of terms is necessary for describing the location of the facility:

- *Hospital based:* located on the main hospital campus;
- *Satellite:* located off the hospital campus.

Two meanings and interpretations are ascribed to *freestanding ambulatory surgery centers.* To some health industry observers, "freestanding" refers to a facility that is physically separate from another health facility, such as a hospital. No reference to governance or linkage to other organizations of the facility or program is implied. In this interpretation of the term, hospitals as well as other providers of health services can sponsor or manage the freestanding ambulatory surgery center.

In the second interpretation of the term, "freestanding" means both a physically separate facility and a facility and program corporately and legally distinct from any other organization. In this sense, by definition all freestanding ambulatory surgery centers are physically separate and organizationally distinct from hospitals. The first interpretation of the term is used here.

In summary, a freestanding ambulatory surgery center connotes a facility physically separate from an inpatient acute care facility. However, the freestanding ambulatory surgery center may vary according to governance structures, types of ownership and sponsorship, comprehensiveness of services, and types of affiliation with hospitals.

DEVELOPMENT

Reasons for Hospital Involvement

There are various reasons why hospital services are expanded or modified to include an ambulatory surgery program. In general, advances in technology that have transformed services delivered to hospitalized inpatients have also transformed the patterns of medical practice and services delivered to ambulatory patients.

The same factors, moreover, that allow for the establishment or operation of other ambulatory care programs in hospitals may be relevant to the decisions made concerning ambulatory surgery. These reasons include changing demand for health services; demographic changes; advent of or increase in competition among providers; preferences of third-party payers and regulators; economies of scale and scope; and corporate objectives of the institutions.[3]

Empirical Evidence

To date, little empirical work has been conducted on the prevalence of ambulatory surgery programs in the United States. In the American Hospital Association (AHA) *1980 Survey of Hospital Involvement with Ambulatory Surgery,* the first data was collected on hospital involvement in the provision of ambulatory surgery.[4] The purpose of the survey was to determine which hospitals were offering ambulatory surgery services, the volume of procedures performed, and the type of facility used. Analysts aimed to gain perspective on hospital involvement in ambulatory surgery. Since that survey was conducted, the AHA Annual Survey of Hospitals was expanded, and the 1980 AHA Annual Survey provides the first nationwide hospital data. Each survey will be discussed in turn.

Survey of Hospital Involvement in Ambulatory Surgery

The survey was mailed to all nonfederal hospitals in the 134 largest U.S. Standard Metropolitan Statistical Areas (SMSAs). Out of a possible 2,955 hospitals, there was a response from 2,137, yielding a response rate of

72.3 percent. Hospitals surveyed included only those located within SMSAs. Although the hospitals surveyed represent approximately half of the hospitals in the United States (50.6 percent), it cannot be assumed that non-SMSA hospitals or hospitals located in small SMSAs that were not in the sample behave similary to those hospitals surveyed.

Of the hospitals surveyed, 70 percent (1,506) offer ambulatory surgical services. Table 1–1 displays the distribution of hospitals, by ownership, that offer ambulatory surgery. Except in very small hospitals (fewer than 100 beds), ambulatory surgery appears to be widespread in hospitals in all bed-size classifications. At least 69 percent of all hospitals in each bed-size category above 100 beds offers ambulatory surgery.

Ambulatory surgery is widespread among types and sizes of hospitals throughout the United States. By geographical area, hospitals performing ambulatory surgery are most prevalent in the East North Central region (Illinois, Indiana, Michigan, Ohio, and Wisconsin). Of hospitals performing ambulatory surgery, 20 percent are located in this region. Similarly, 19 percent of the hospitals are located in the Middle Atlantic region (New Jersey, New York, and Pennsylvania), and 18 percent are located in the Pacific region (Arkansas, California, Hawaii, Oregon, and Washington). Of the hospitals performing ambulatory surgery, 15 percent are in California and 8 percent are in Pennsylvania.

Although only 4 percent of the hospitals performing ambulatory surgery are in the Mountain region (Arizona, Colorado, Idaho, Missouri, Nevada, New Mexico, Utah, and Wyoming), these 59 hospitals represent 80 percent of the hospitals in that region.

Organized Programs. Although 70 percent of the hospitals surveyed reported that they perform ambulatory surgery, only 54 percent of these, or 803 hospitals, have organized ambulatory surgery programs. (See Table 1–2 for distribution of organized ambulatory surgery programs by type.) This figure represents 38 percent of all hospitals surveyed. There appears to be more of a tendency for a hospital to organize its program as the hospital bed size increases, although 43 percent of the hospitals having between 100 and 199 beds do have an organized ambulatory surgery program.

By type of ownership, only 39 percent of the for-profit hospitals with ambulatory surgery have organized programs, whereas 57 percent of the not-for-profit hospitals have organized ambulatory surgery programs. This difference could be more a result of size than ownership because the for-profit hospitals are generally small. At any rate, 79 percent of all organized ambulatory surgery programs are located in not-for-profit hospitals—20 percent in church-related hospitals and 59 percent in other not-for-profit

Table 1-1 Facility Used for Ambulatory Surgery in Hospitals in 134 Largest SMSAs by Bed Size and Ownership in the United States, 1980

Hospital	Hospitals Offering Ambulatory Surgery		Inpatient and Ambulatory	Exclusively Ambulatory near Inpatient	Separate within Hospital Complex	Separate from Inpatient Hospital	Other
	Number	Percentage	Percentage	Percentage	Percentage	Percentage	Percentage
Nonfederal							
less than 25 beds	11	39.3	90.9	0	0	0	0
25–49 beds	57	37.7	96.5	3.5	3.5	1.8	1.8
50–99 beds	157	46.7	95.5	5.1	1.3	.6	3.8
100–199 beds	395	70.8	91.6	5.3	7.3	.8	3.0
200–299 beds	300	83.6	85.7	8.7	13.3	2.0	6.3
300–399 beds	227	86.0	83.3	11.9	14.1	1.8	6.6
400–499 beds	142	89.3	81.0	12.7	16.9	4.9	4.2
500 or more beds	217	77.0	75.1	17.5	28.6	5.5	5.5
Total	1,506	70.5	86.4	9.3	12.7	2.3	4.7
Not for profit	1,107	79.7	85.3	10.2	12.8	2.4	5.2
Church related	281	86.5	83.3	11.7	14.9	1.8	5.7
Other	826	77.6	86.0	9.7	12.1	2.7	5.1
For profit	180	55.4	93.3	5.0	6.7	1.1	.6
State and local government	219	51.8	86.3	8.2	16.9	2.3	5.5

Source: American Hospital Association, 1980 Survey of Hospital Involvement with Ambulatory Surgery.

Table 1-2 Percentage and Number of Hospitals Operating
Ambulatory Surgery Programs in the 134 Largest SMSAs
in the United States, 1980

Hospitals	Offer Ambulatory Surgery		Offer Organized Ambulatory Surgery Program	
	Number	Percentage	Number	Percentage
Nonfederal	1,506	70.5	805	53.5
Not for profit	1,107	79.7	634	57.3
Church related	281	86.5	161	57.3
Other	826	77.6	473	57.3
For profit	180	55.4	71	39.4
State and local government	219	51.8	100	45.7

Source: American Hospital Association, *1980 Survey of Hospital Involvement with Ambulatory Surgery.*

hospitals. Only 9 percent of all organized ambulatory surgery programs are located in for-profit hospitals. State and local government hospitals account for 12 percent of the organized programs.

The geographical location of *organized* ambulatory surgery programs does not differ substantially from that of hospitals with *any* ambulatory surgery. In each state in which hospitals offer some type of ambulatory surgery, there is at least one organized ambulatory surgery program. California has 108 hospitals with organized ambulatory surgery programs; this figure represents half of the total number of hospitals in the state with ambulatory surgery and 36 percent of the hospitals in the state. Pennsylvania also has a high number of hospitals (84) with organized programs.

By region, 22 percent of the organized programs are in the Middle Atlantic region. They are found in 60 percent of the hospitals with ambulatory surgery in Middle Atlantic states. Nineteen percent of the programs are in the East North Central region, representing 50 percent of the hospitals with ambulatory surgery in that area.

Degree of Commitment. Some judgment as to the commitment to and prevalence of ambulatory surgery can be made by observing the type of surgical facility used. In other words, does the hospital simply use the existing operating suites for inpatient and ambulatory surgery; or are there separate operating suites exclusively for ambulatory surgery near the inpatient suites, separate from the inpatient suites but within the hospital complex, or freestanding from the hospital? Of relevance to hospital decision makers is the question of whether the hospital faces excessive demand for surgery or inpatient beds. Table 1–1 also presents the facility arrangements used by hospitals that offer ambulatory surgery by bed size and hospital ownership.

Of the 1,506 hospitals offering ambulatory surgery, 87 percent use the main operating suites for inpatient and ambulatory surgery. This arrangement is directly related to the size of the hospitals, ranging from all hospitals under 25 beds to 75 percent of the hospitals over 500 beds. As bed size increases there is more of a tendency to use separate facilities exclusively for ambulatory surgery, but this phenomenon is not common.

By hospital ownership, the for-profit hospitals appear to be least likely to dedicate separate facilities of any kind to ambulatory surgery. Again, this tendency could be a factor of the small size of the average for-profit hospital rather than of its for-profit characteristic. Proportionally, the mountain region has more separate facilities, both hospital based and freestanding, than any other region in the United States.

Surgery Centers. Ambulatory surgery is also provided in settings—often known as "surgery centers"—independent of hospitals. Of the hospitals responding to the AHA survey, 592, or 28 percent, reported knowledge of an ambulatory surgery center independent of their hospital governance and physically separate from the hospital facility in their service areas.

The largest number of hospitals with freestanding, independent ambulatory surgery centers in their service areas is found in California. Ninety-two California hospitals believe that there is an independent surgery center in their service areas. This area is followed by Texas, where there are 40 hospitals with independent surgery centers in their service areas, then by Pennsylvania and Florida, each with 34.

Revenues. The average annual number of ambulatory surgical procedures performed in 1979 was reported as 1,245 per hospital as compared with 5,649 inpatient procedures. Due to the fact that ambulatory surgery consumes a less costly mix of inputs because of the less complicated nature of the surgical procedures than major inpatient operations, the amount of revenue per case derived from ambulatory surgery is less than the revenue per case derived from inpatient surgery. The assumption might be that prices for surgery correlate with costs of production. In fact, in the hospitals surveyed, ambulatory surgery accounted for only 8 percent of total surgical revenue in 1979, whereas it accounted for 18 percent of total surgical procedures. Gross revenues for surgical procedures performed in hospitals with ambulatory surgery programs for fiscal year 1979 are displayed in Table 1–3.

Table 1-3 Gross Revenues for Surgical Procedures Performed in Hospitals with Ambulatory Surgery Programs in the 134 Largest SMSAs by Bed Size and Ownership in the United States, Fiscal 1979

Hospitals	Hospitals Offering Ambulatory Surgery (Number)	All Surgery Revenues ($000)	Ambulatory Surgery Revenues ($000)
Nonfederal hospitals			
less than 25 beds	11	936.3	249.0
25–49 beds	57	9,712.1	1,024.0
50–99 beds	157	56,126.2	4,537.6
100–199 beds	395	301,127.9	32,790.3
200–299 beds	300	443,620.9	29,474.0
300–399 beds	227	495,679.2	34,166.1
400–499 beds	142	383,456.7	28,211.6
500 or more beds	217	978,262.8	62,956.0
Total	1,506	2,688,922.1	193,408.6
Not for profit	1,107	2,180,190.8	158,061.2
Church related	281	626,483.5	44,312.1
Other	826	1,553,707.3	113,749.1
For profit	180	122,851.6	18,949.6
State and local government	219	365,879.7	16,397.8

Source: American Hospital Association, *1980 Survey of Hospital Involvement with Ambulatory Surgery.*

1980 Annual Survey of Hospitals

The AHA Annual Survey was expanded, and data has been collected for fiscal year 1980 regarding hospital ambulatory surgery programs. Data was collected from all general hospitals in the United States. These statistics comprise the first and most comprehensive nationwide data on hospital ambulatory surgery programs.

Table 1–4 shows that nationwide 66.4 percent of the hospitals provide ambulatory surgical services; 73.9 percent of the hospitals located in SMSAs offer ambulatory surgery, while 58.0 percent of the hospitals located in non-SMSAs offer ambulatory surgery. In Table 1–5 ambulatory surgery is given as a percentage of total surgery in hospitals by bed size. Small hospitals perform proportionately more ambulatory surgery than do larger hospitals. Table 1–6 lists hospitals by region and shows the proportion of ambulatory surgery to total surgery for each. By region, hospitals in the New England, Mountain, and Pacific regions perform more of their surgery on an ambulatory basis than hospitals in other regions of the United States.

Table 1-4 Hospitals Offering Ambulatory Surgery in U.S. Standard Metropolitan Statistical Areas (SMSAs), 1980

Category	Number of Hospitals	Hospitals Offering Ambulatory Surgery	Percentage of Total
All hospitals	6,370	4,228	66.4
SMSA	3,342	2,471	73.9
Non-SMSA	3,028	1,757	58.0

Source: American Hospital Association 1980 Annual Survey of Hospitals.

Table 1-5 Ambulatory Surgery as a Percentage of Total Surgery in U.S. Hospitals by Bed Size, 1980

Category	Number of Hospitals	Total Surgical Procedures	Ambulatory Procedures (Percentage of Total)
All hospitals	6,370	19,602,964	16.4
6–24 beds	294	64,129	30.8
25–49	1,124	425,110	16.0
50–99	1,525	1,513,595	22.7
100–199	1,453	3,725,842	15.4
200–299	757	3,775,503	16.7
300–399	455	3,141,064	17.8
400–499	302	2,547,737	16.5
500 or more	460	4,409,984	15.1

Source: American Hospital Association 1980 Annual Survey of Hospitals.

Table 1–7 reveals that 66.4 percent of hospitals nationwide offer ambulatory surgery and shows the distribution of hospitals by type of control. The data reveals that nongovernment not-for-profit hospitals provide proportionately more ambulatory surgery than other types of hospitals.

The data in these tables confirms the initial data from the 1980 Special Survey. In addition, it further establishes that hospitals located in non-SMSAs and federal hospitals provide ambulatory surgical services to the same extent as other hospitals.

FREESTANDING INDEPENDENT CENTERS

The Dudley Street Ambulatory Surgical Center in Providence, Rhode Island, the first freestanding, independent surgical center documented, was opened in December 1968 by Charles Hill and his associates. In

Table 1-6 Ambulatory Surgery As a Percentage of Total Surgery in
U.S. Hospitals by Region, 1980

Category	Number of Hospitals	Total Surgical Procedures	Ambulatory Procedures (Percentage of Total)
All hospitals	6,370	19,602,964	16.4
New England	303	1,078,331	22.0
Middle Atlantic	685	3,187,390	19.5
South Atlantic	928	3,201,427	16.3
East North Central	970	3,821,783	17.9
East South Central	528	1,329,423	13.1
West North Central	851	1,658,099	15.5
West South Central	900	2,052,500	11.2
Mountain	409	914,406	19.4
Pacific	796	1,359,605	18.3

Source: American Hospital Association 1980 Annual Survey of Hospitals.

Table 1-7 Number of U.S. Hospitals Offering Ambulatory Surgery
Services by Governance, 1980

Category	Total Number of Hospitals	Hospitals with Ambulatory Surgery	Percentage of Total
All hospitals	6,370	4,288	66.4
Government (nonfederal)	1,937	1,031	53.2
Nongovernment (not for profit)	3,330	2,578	77.4
Nongovernment (for profit)	775	414	53.4
Government (federal)	332	205	63.7

Source: American Hospital Association 1980 Annual Survey of Hospitals.

February 1970 the well-known Surgicenter® in Phoenix, Arizona, was established by anesthesiologists Wallace Reed and John Ford.

The success of the Phoenix center precipitated rapid growth of a new type of facility for the delivery of ambulatory surgery—the freestanding, independent ambulatory surgery center. Since that time, the Surgicenter® has become a model for an increasing number of both independent and hospital-sponsored freestanding ambulatory surgical centers. Often its name is used generically to describe ambulatory surgery programs.

According to the Freestanding Ambulatory Surgical Association (FASA), there are approximately 125 independent freestanding ambulatory surgery centers, 86 of which are members of FASA. According to FASA, which has been keeping statistics on its members since 1974, the membership

Table 1-8 Ten Most Common Ambulatory Surgery Procedures in Independent Freestanding Centers, 1981

Procedure	Percentage of Total Procedures
Dilatation and curettage	14.9
Laparoscopy	11.5
Orthopedic procedures	10.4
Myringotomy	9.6
Excision of mass/skin lesion	8.6
Arthroscopy	4.3
Tonsillectomy and/or adenoidectomy	3.9
Dental procedures	3.4
Plastic procedures	3.2
Cystoscopy	2.0
Total	72.2

Source: Freestanding Ambulatory Surgical Association, Eighth Annual Meeting, April 1, 1982.

performed 94,499 ambulatory surgery procedures in 1981, an increase of 6 percent over the number performed in 1980. This figure can be compared to 3.2 million ambulatory surgical procedures performed by hospitals offering ambulatory surgery in 1980.

Of the procedures performed at the independent facilities, 72 percent requested the use of general anesthesia, 3 percent used conduction, and 25 percent used either local or no anesthesia. No deaths were reported by any of the facilities in 1981. Ten procedures accounted for over 72 percent of the total ambulatory surgery performed in the independent facilities. (See Table 1-8.) Published data is unavailable regarding geographical dispersion of independent surgery centers, source of patients by payer, staffing, revenues, and costs.

PUBLIC POLICY ISSUES

Several important public policy issues emerge as a result of the growth of ambulatory surgery programs. These issues involve accreditation, licensure, health system agency review, legal concerns, and reimbursement policies.

Accreditation

The Joint Commission on Accreditation of Hospitals (JCAH), in its *1981 Accreditation Manual for Hospitals,* specifies the following:

When surgical services are provided in an ambulatory care setting, the policies and procedures shall be consistent with those applicable to inpatient surgery, anesthesia, and post-operative recovery, and shall address, in addition to the preceding policies and procedures, the following:

- Types of elective operative procedures that may be performed and the locations where they may be performed.
- Scope of anesthesia services that may be provided and the locations where such anesthesia services may be administered.
- Preoperative and postoperative transportation.
- An established method of intervention when the designated preoperative patient workup and preparation are incomplete. An operation shall be performed only after an appropriate history, physical examination, and any required laboratory and x-ray examinations have been completed and the preoperative diagnosis has been recorded.
- Postoperative care, including postanesthesia recovery patient care guidelines and the role of family members assisting in patient care. Any patient who has received other than local anesthesia shall be examined by a qualified physician before discharge and shall be accompanied home by a designated person. Written instructions for follow-up care shall be given to the patient or responsible family member, and shall include directions for obtaining appropriate physician help in the event of postoperative problems. Whenever feasible, a family member should be available to pediatric patients during the preoperative and postoperative periods.[5]

The JCAH can accredit freestanding ambulatory surgery centers that are not governed by hospitals. The JCAH operates an Ambulatory Health Care Accreditation Program in addition to a Hospital Accreditation program. Although the JCAH has accredited several independent surgery centers, in 1980 JCAH surveyors reported that no JCAH surveys were conducted for independent ambulatory surgery centers.

Currently, Section 934 of the Omnibus Reconciliation Act of 1980 proposes that deemed status for Medicare certification be provided to a voluntary accreditation body. The Accreditation Association for Ambulatory Health Care (AAAHC)—established in 1979 and independent of JCAH—

accredited 40 freestanding, independent ambulatory surgery centers. The FASA is a charter member of AAAHC.

Licensure

The issue of state licensure has been approached in various ways. Hospital-sponsored and hospital-associated facilities generally fall under the state hospital facility survey and licensing authority, whereas independent, freestanding ambulatory surgery centers have largely been overlooked by individual states. Private physicians who operate independent, freestanding ambulatory surgery centers have maintained that they are already licensed to practice medicine and therefore require no additional licensure; they claim the ambulatory surgery center essentially represents their private practice office.

Health Systems Agency Review

Under the Health Planning and Resources Development Act of 1974 (PL 93–641) and its subsequent amendments, state governments are supposed to establish certificate-of-need (CON) programs to regulate significant changes in health care facilities and services. Under the separation of powers established by the U.S. Constitution, the establishment of hospitals and other health facilities is a state rather than a federal responsibility; consequently, PL 93–641 assigned the law's CON functions to the states. As of 1982, most states had complied with this mandate.

The basic structure of CON reviews is founded on earlier CON statutes in states such as New York, which established the principles of having local areawide health planning agencies provide recommendations to the state agency as to whether a particular health care facility project should be approved. Under PL 93–641, an areawide agency is called a Health Systems Agency (HSA); state CON programs are required to seek the advice of the HSA if there is one.

Legal Concerns

Hospitals and other entities that are considering establishing ambulatory surgery programs should ascertain whether the state's CON program requires state approval, and, if so, whether there is an HSA (or other local agency) whose review is mandated under the CON process. In several states where the law particularly reflects federal details, a CON may be required for a project if it is sponsored by a hospital but not if it is sponsored by another entity. Under this circumstance, hospitals would be regulated and other facilities would not. This distinction may have promoted the unfortunate reluctance of community hospitals to establish ambulatory surgery programs, because they know they would be faced with an expensive and slow process in obtaining a CON while other facilities could develop competing projects without being subject to the regulations imposed on hospitals.

Many states exempt facilities from the CON process if they can be classified as physician's offices rather than licensed institutions. It should be noted, however, that in some jurisdictions, a facility that charges for institutional services may not be able to qualify as a surgeon's private office. The laws and regulations regarding this distinction are fluid at both the federal and state levels, particularly in light of the present popularity of deregulation.

Regardless of whether there is a legal requirement for CON review, sponsors are usually well advised to share their ambulatory surgery plans with the local HSA, if there is one, or with whatever other agency has assumed the areawide health planning role if the HSA has ceased to function or if there is no HSA.

Reimbursement Policies

There are two components of the total charge for a surgical procedure. One component—the facility fee —is the cost of the technical resources used in performing the surgical procedure such as the surgical suite, operating room nursing staff, and supplies. The second component is the charge for the physician's professional services. Various third party payers have established reimbursement and payment policies regarding these two components. Although policies vary among types of payers and among specific insurers and fiscal intermediaries, some general provisions can be identified.

Section 934 of Title IX of the Omnibus Reconciliation Act of 1980 (PL 96–499) addresses the Medicare provisions concerning ambulatory surgery and changes previously enacted legislation pertaining to ambulatory surgery. According to Section 934, physicians' professional services will be reimbursed at 100 percent of reasonable charges for surgery performed in an ambulatory rather than an inpatient setting; such reimbursement will be subject to the conditions in the Act, including acceptance of assignment by the physician. Physicans performing surgery on an inpatient basis will continue to be reimbursed at 80 percent of reasonable charges. In addition, the Act allows independent ambulatory surgery centers to be reimbursed for the first time for facility charges.

According to proposed rules published in the March 23, 1982, *Federal Register* and developed to implement the Act, independent ambulatory surgery centers will be paid a prospectivley determined facility fee to cover the technical component of the total charge for an ambulatory surgical procedure. Medicare payment will be made at 100 percent of the established rate per procedure. There will be no beneficiary liability for coinsurnace on the Part B deductible. Section 934 made no changes in the reimbursement policy for facility costs associated with hospital-sponsored or hospital-associated ambulatory surgery programs. The costs will continue to be included in the hospital's Medicare cost reports and reimbursed at the reasonable cost level. Medicare beneficiary deductible and coinsurance amounts will still apply. This results in potential competitive advantages to the nonhospital providers of ambulatory surgery for Medicare patients.

Each Blue Cross and Blue Shield plan determines its own reimbursement and payment policies for ambulatory surgery. However, some idea of the associations' policies can be derived from examining the policies of their national trade association. According to a January 1981 policy issued by the Blue Cross and Blue Shield Associations:

> The policy of the Blue Cross and Blue Shield Associations and their member plans is that surgery, like any other health care service, should be performed in the least costly manner enabling delivery of safe high quality patient care. To achieve this goal, the Associations and plans encourage both appropriate growth of ambulatory surgery and more selective use of inpatient care for surgery.[6]

The Blue Cross and Blue Shield Associations caution, however, that "shifts in the location of surgery from physician offices to more costly hospital outpatient or freestanding facility settings need to be monitored. Changes in hospital costs that might be attributed to shifts in surgery settings need to be monitored as well."[6] The Associations are urging Blue Cross and Blue Shield plans to fashion incentives to providers and consumers "to have surgery done where it can be most appropriately and efficiently performed."[6]

Reimbursement policies by commercial insurance carriers vary by company. In general, the commercial insurance carriers are charge-based payers. Reimbursable charges are based on a percentage of usual and customary rates. The Health Insurance Association of America regards ambulatory surgery as a cost-saving program and recommends that insurance plans cover ambulatory surgical services provided by licensed physicians in a recognized establishment, whether hospital sponsored or not, in the same manner that they reimburse other surgical services.

Scale or Scope. There are at least two aspects of the organizational arrangement of ambulatory surgery programs that are likely to affect the cost of care and that relate to the policy choices of interest to both the industry and third party payers, including the government. The issues are economies of *scale* (i.e., whether costs per unit of service decline as the size of the ambulatory surgery center increases) and economies of *scope* (i.e., whether ambulatory services are produced more inexpensively in combination with other hospital services or in separate physician offices).

Health services research has not adequately investigated these issues. The 1977 Orkand Corporation effort, for example—"Comparative Evaluation of Costs, Quality, and System Effects of Ambulatory Surgery Performed in Alternative Settings"—attempted to compare production costs among types of ambulatory surgery providers.[7] The results, however, were inconclusive because of the dilemma of accounting for indirect costs.

Joint costs are those production costs associated with more than one output. In a hospital that produces both inpatient and ambulatory surgery, for example, there are costs associated with administration that are properly chargeable to no specific output but must be accounted for. Single output firms, such as independent, freestanding ambulatory surgery centers, do not face the dilemma of joint costs; therefore, their production costs are easily measured. Hospitals, on the other hand, employ cost allocation methodologies that are arbitrary and that mask their true production costs.

Ambulatory surgery programs represent an alternative way of organizing and delivering health services. Critical questions concerning the benefits and costs to society of these developments must be explored further. At a minimum, current regulatory and reimbursement policies should not create perverse incentives to providers to organize ambulatory surgery and other health services in ways that result in greater costs than benefits to the public.

REFERENCES

1. American Hospital Association: *Hospital Statistics*. Chicago, American Hospital Association, 1981, p 5.
2. Burns LA, Ferber MS: Definitions proposed for hospital roles in ambulatory care. *Outreach* 1980;1 (August):2–4.
3. Burns, LA: Will multi-institutional systems serve as change agents to improve the management of ambulatory care? *JACM* 1980;3 (August):1–17.
4. American Hospital Association. *1980 Survey of Hospital Involvement with Ambulatory Surgery*. Chicago, American Hospital Association, 1980.

5. Joint Commission on Accreditation of Hospitals: *Accreditation Manual for Hospitals*. Chicago, Joint Commission on Accreditation of Hospitals, 1981, p 66.

6. Blue Cross and Blue Shield Associations: *Policy and Recommendations of the Blue Cross and Blue Shield Associations on Ambulatory Surgery*. Chicago, Blue Cross and Blue Shield Associations, 1981, pp 1–2.

7. The Orkand Corporation: *Comparative Evaluation of Costs, Quality and System Effects of Ambulatory Surgery Performed in Alternative Settings*, US DHEW Health Care Financing Administration, December 1977.

Chapter 2

Marketing Ambulatory Surgery Centers: Planning Considerations and Demand Analysis

Eric N. Berkowitz, Ph.D.

The growth of ambulatory care facilities has been well documented, but though evidence of ambulatory surgery before World War II exists, it is only in recent years that the shift toward ambulatory surgery has become noticeable.[1] As a result of this change and the increasingly competitive environment of health care providers, many organizations are considering ambulatory surgery centers to improve their stategic position. Development of such facilities requires marketing plans and prior market analysis.

Effective marketing planning for an ambulatory surgery center requires several basic elements: (1) an understanding of the nature of marketing (although this need may seem obvious, the marketing concept is still new to health care); (2) an understanding of the macroenvironment in which the plans will be developed, and the marketing implications of any discernible trends; (3) recognition of who the consumers are and what they want; (4) recognition or attention to the uniqueness of the organization's facility relative to the competition; and (5) assessment of the demand for the ambulatory surgery center.

A MARKETING ORIENTATION

Marketing has received much attention in recent years in health care management literature.[2] In discussing marketing, it is essential to recognize that a marketing focus begins with the consumer. The wants and needs of the market are assessed, and a service is developed to meet these needs. Marketing is not selling, but selling is a component of effective marketing. An example from one ambulatory care facility may clarify this distinction.

Adapted from *Journal of Ambulatory Care Management* 1981;3:1–13.

A large not-for-profit hospital in a major metropolitan area recently opened an ambulatory care facility. No prior analysis was conducted to determine the need for such a service among any particular group. Contracts were signed with several physicians to provide specific services in sports medicine, executive fitness, and the like. As the facility's opening date approached, the administration was concerned as to the level of use by physicians and the public. A marketing consultant was hired as well as an in-house director of marketing. Their task was to develop marketing plans.

At this stage of the scenario, the task is actually to develop a sales program. The sales situation is indicated in Table 2–1, showing a fixed facility with decided-on products, personnel, and, most important, costs. The primary goal for the organization is to develop usage levels. A marketing orientation also is shown in Table 2–1. First, prospective user groups are identified and the needs assessed. An assessment of demand is made and, if favorable, a program is developed. In the final phase the program is promoted to the respective user groups. The role of marketing vis-à-vis selling has been highlighted best by Drucker: "The aim of marketing is to make selling superfluous. The aim of marketing is to know and understand the consumer so well that the product or service fits him and sells itself."[3]

In the most effective and efficient marketing system, the only sales task would be to inform prospective users that their need had been satisfied. Understanding this flow implies that before an organization decides to build an ambulatory care facility, an external market analysis is conducted.

Table 2-1 Sales versus Marketing Orientation

Condition	Sales Perspective Mission		Goal
Fixed facility personnel service mix	→	Develop informational programs for prospective users	→ Obtain utilization

Condition	Marketing Perspective Mission	Goal	Task
Interest in program by organization	→ Define users; assess demand	→ Meet market need	→ Develop informational programs for prospective users

PLANNING ENVIRONMENT

Accepting a marketing philosophy is not sufficient for successful marketing plans. Figure 2–1 displays the several elements in the macroenvironment that must be monitored.

Mounting Costs and Controls

The increasing cost of health care has been cited often. And as health care becomes an increasingly larger proportion of the U.S. Gross National Product (GNP), the industry will become more visible. Present estimates indicate 8.5 percent of the GNP is devoted to health care.[4] As health care dollars or company benefit packages take a larger percentage of the consumers' income, costs may become a major criterion in the selection of alternative care sources. In this respect consumer acceptance of ambulatory surgery may be more likely in that a real cost savings can be promoted.[5] Moreover, companies may show greater interest in this alternative as a way to reduce health coverage costs.

Figure 2–1 Environmental Considerations for Effective Marketing Strategy

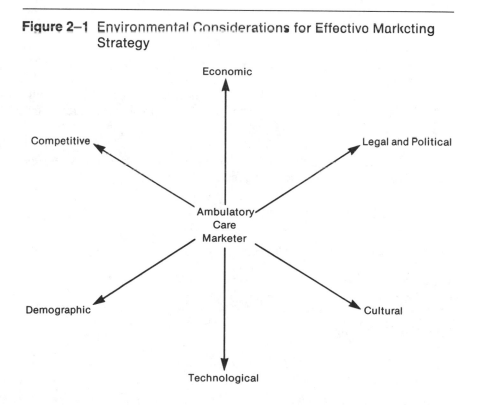

Regulatory Changes

Nowhere in the macro planning environment have more changes occurred of late than in the legal area. The legal dimension has been felt on the local and federal levels. Health Systems Agency Network (HSA) created by PL 93–641 changed the control any health provider has over its own destiny. Yet the magnitude of these legal changes may be just beginning. A new administration in Washington, D.C., has shifted to a deregulated, competitive position. In March 1980 David Clanton, chairman of the Federal Trade Commission, discussed the priorities of his agency under the Reagan Administration. He noted that emphasis will be

> on particularly troublesome kinds of behavior; such as attempts by those who provide health care to obstruct cost containment programs through price fixing or boycotts. . . . Competition can play a significant role in helping to relieve [the] inflationary pressures of spiraling health care costs.[6]

Consumer Challenges

The attitudes of consumers toward life, life styles, and the institutions with which they interact have changed considerably in recent years. These changes have been reflected in the use of day-care centers, natural foods, generic drugs, and the like. At the St. Louis University Medical Center, Virginia Knauer, a former special assistant to the president for consumer affairs, recently cited the following:

- In one survey, 25 percent of the respondents felt that hospitals and the medical profession do a "poor" job.
- Consumers can be expected to question such details as dosage, length of treatment, and side effects.
- Consumers are challenging and will continue to challenge surgical recommendations.[7]

These changes portray a new, more critical attitude toward the health care provider and the heatlh care system in general.

Changing Technology

There is little need to discuss the technological changes that have occurred and are occurring in health care. Yet this high technology places the physician and administrator in a difficult position. Consumers are aware of computer-assisted technology such as CAT scanners and other sophisticated forms of diagnosis. Technology, then, does one thing to consumers: It raises their expectation level. The likelihood of a dissatisfied patient is greater now, because every consumer *expects* to be cured. Consumers no longer want only good care; they believe they should receive sophisticated, high-technology service.

Shifting Market

Effective marketing requires a fine tuning to demographic shifts. The present location of many hospitals was once in the midst of a very different sociodemographic market area. Just as department stores have followed their customers to the suburbs by locating in shopping malls, some hospitals have responded with satellite clinics. One hospital in Chicago responded to the area's demographics by providing a day-care center for the elderly.[8] (No research was conducted among the elderly consumers themselves, however, and the service was not successful upon introduction.) Future facility planners must consider the inclusion of services that will reflect the usage pattern not only of their existing patient population but also of the forecasted profile of future residents.

Increasing Competition

The competitive environment of health care is changing rapidly. Most administrators now readily admit that they compete with each other. Ambulatory surgery centers, freestanding emergency centers, medi-vans, and health maintenance organizations (HMOs) are only a few of the more recent competitive influences. There is some indication that greater competition does reduce costs.[9] This increasingly competitive environment makes it more difficult to manage a successful organization. Monitoring these macrodimensions alone will not result in successful marketing plans. A basic factor in effective planning is to identify who the consumers are and what they need.

MULTIPLE CONSUMERS AND DIFFERING NEEDS

Developing plans for an ambulatory surgery facility is often difficult because of the multiple markets or publics that might have to be considered. Figure 2–2 indicates several such groups. A major difficulty in health marketing is this multiplicity of publics who often have very differing

Figure 2-2 Multiple Market Base for Ambulatory Surgery Facility

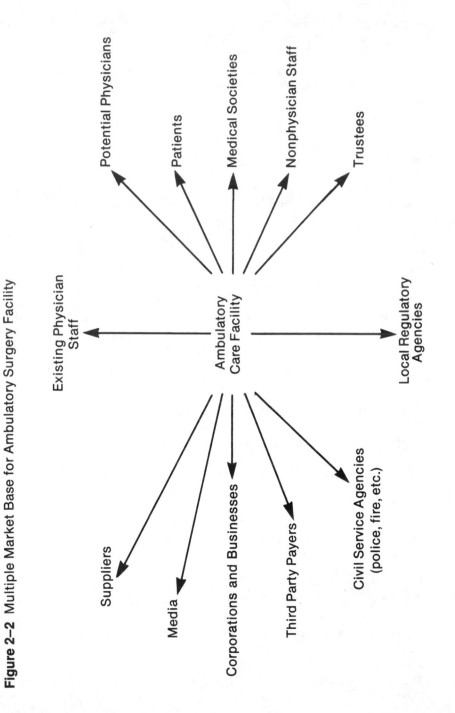

needs. Each group has a different definition of what an ambulatory surgical center should provide.

Physician's Perspective

The success of any ambulatory surgery center is particularly dependent on the staff physicians. As with the marketing of most "high-contact" services, the quality of the health care service cannot be defined apart from the quality of the service provider.[10] As Berry has indicated, "service marketers need to be concerned with service quality, which means in labor-intensive situations—special attention to employee quality and performance."[11] For the administrator of an ambulatory surgery center, an internal marketing strategy must consider these staff members as customers, and the service must be designed to meet their needs most efficiently. At a recent ambulatory surgery conference sponsored by the AMA, an administrator related this scenario:

> We opened an elaborate ambulatory surgery center last year. However, in spite of rather extensive promotional efforts, the use of the facility is well below projections. The surgery center is located in a separate building across the parking lot from the hospital. The physicians did not use the center because they did not want to walk across the lot.

The location of this facility did not meet the physicians' needs in terms of convenience. They did not see the benefit of scheduling procedures at this site when all surgical needs could be met at one location. At present the administrator is considering buying electric golf carts to transport physicians between facilities. This example portrays a costly lack of prior consideration of user needs.

Patients' Perspective

It is essential to understand that every group will define the product differently. Patients define ambulatory surgery differently than physicians. As Figure 2–3 shows, the patients' view of the health care product consists of a generic product and an offered product. The *generic product* refers to the class of services provided—in this case the medical technology provided by the physician at the surgical center. Yet the variations of the generic product are only discernible to other trained providers of the service. The offered product includes several of the elements reviewed by Kovner and Smits.[12] These components include facility ambience, con-

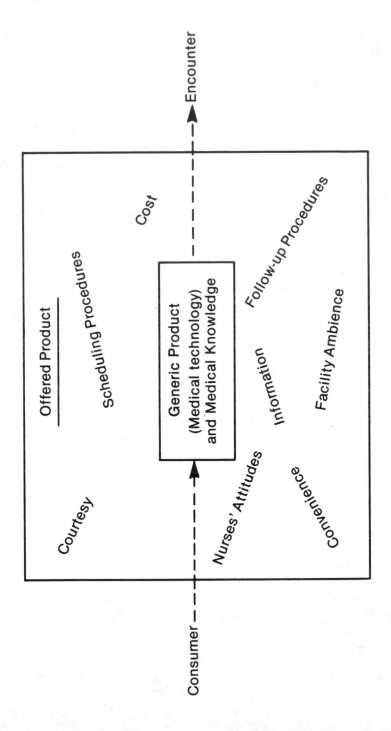

Figure 2–3 Consumer Definition of the Health Care Encounter

venience, nurses' attitudes, cost, and follow-up procedures. Thus, the *offered product* pertains to the augmentations of providing the medical knowledge and the medical technology, the generic product.

All these elements may be part of the patients' definition of the care they receive. As a result it is equally important that these other dimensions of the product also be provided in a way that best meets users' needs. Too often the patients' definition is not considered. As Lachner indicates: whether it is the physician, the house staff member or the nurse, the waiter, x-ray, emergency department or the admitting clerk who is rude, the maid who bumps the bed while cleaning, the parking lot attendant who is less than helpful when the lot is full, the cafeteria that turns away visitors, the pharmacy that has limited hours for outpatients—all of this suggests that hospitals operate for their own convenience and not that of the patient, family and friends.[13]

Although defining the product from the users' view may seem easy, it is difficult to operationalize. Examples from two existing ambulatory surgery centers may illustrate the problem more clearly.

In the first example, a large hospital in the southwest has a day surgery unit open Monday through Saturday from 6:30 A.M. to 6:00 P.M. On the day before surgery, patients must come to the facility for laboratory tests and to complete admission forms. The following day, patients must report to the day surgery unit at 6:30 A.M. so that they will be available to the attending surgeon and anesthesiologist. This procedure allows patients to be shifted in the schedule flexibly and as need arises. Surgery procedures are scheduled up to 2:00 P.M.

In the second example, a similar facility in the Northwest also performs surgery from early morning to midafternoon. This organization has developed a multimedia presentation to describe the ambulatory surgery procedures to prospective patients. Two versions of the presentation have been created—one for adults and one for children. Prospective patients come to the facility the day before surgery to view the presentation and to complete the admission forms. Whenever possible, laboratory tests are conducted on the day of surgery.

Each of these examples should be viewed from the patients' perspective to determine whether the service meets their needs. Both facilities provide excellent care on the generic level, and, to a greater extent, many dimensions of the offered product are highly satisfactory. In the first example, however, patients who may be scheduled for surgery at noon must report to the unit 4½ hours earlier. Convenience for the patients does not seem to be of primary importance. Moreover, on the preceding day, patients must come to the facility to fill out admission forms. For individuals who must drive any distance, the day-before-visit requirement and the early-morning arrival time may involve staying in a hotel, which is not covered by insurance. One can envision a patient opting for inpatient care, because it is more convenient and lower in out-of-pocket costs. To provide a better offered product, admission forms could be mailed to the patient or filled out by telephone. Scheduling systems could be developed to reduce waiting time on the day of surgery.

In the second example, the organization recognizes that there are different segments of the patient market—adults and children. As a result, separate informational programs have been developed for each group. An even better strategy might be to bring the presentation to the consumer. The presentation and completion of the admission form could be done in the patients' homes, for example, using volunteers or low-cost nonprofessional staff.

The importance of the users' definition of the service cannot be overemphasized. This consideration becomes more important as competition increases, and it is the focus of the fourth factor in developing marketing strategy.

NEED FOR DIFFERENTIAL ADVANTAGE

Increasing interest in the establishment of ambulatory surgical centers already has been noted. This factor, as well as other competitive trends cited earlier, highlights the greater competitive environment in which ambulatory surgery centers will operate. Even if regulatory approval is obtained, the hospital that considers opening the second or third surgery center in an area must attempt to differentiate itself from the competition. The most difficult assessment to be made by an organization is how it differs from competitors; that is, in what way could the offered product better meet the needs of a prospective market?

Consider two surgery centers in relative proximity. One center requires a 6:30 A.M. check-in time regardless of when surgery is scheduled, while the other center requires patients to check in three hours before the scheduled procedure. Differentiation in this instance is obvious. Assuming a patient's physician had surgical privileges at either facility, the location choice could be left with the patient.

Some may believe that health care cannot be differentiated. Levitt has stated, however, that there is no such thing as a commodity and that all goods and services are differentiable. He presented the following example:

> On the commodities exchanges . . . dealers in metals, grains and
> porkbellies trade in totally undifferentiated . . . products. But

what they "sell" is the claimed distinction of their execution—
the efficiency of their transactions in their clients' behalf, their
responsiveness to inquiries, the clarity and speed of their confir-
mations, and the like.[14]

In this situation, the differentiation is developed on the offered rather than
the generic product. Assuming that two ambulatory surgery centers perform the same procedures, there is likely to be little difference in the
generic product being offered; it is through the offered product dimension
that differentiation can be achieved.

NEED FOR SURGERY CENTERS

Two final considerations must be determined before developing specific
marketing strategies: whether a need exists, and the level of the demand
among specific markets. Demand analysis takes two forms—quantitative
and qualitative.

Market research studies typically begin with qualitative research and
follow with quantitative analysis.[15] Demand analysis for ambulatory surgery centers, however, should proceed according to the four stages shown
in Figure 2–4. Initially, internal quantitative analysis should be conducted
by the administration.

Stage 1

Stage 1 should provide initial data to administrators as to whether the
establishment of the facility is justified and worthy of further exploration.
Data for this stage is available from existing records and often can be
obtained without major disruption. Politically this sequence allows the
data to be examined before dealing with the concerns of respective markets, such as physicians or regulatory agencies.

At this stage, such factors as physician demand should be explored.
This analysis should review data on surgical procedures performed for the
preceding five years. Although a five-year period is not a specific requirement, trend data of a reasonable time period should be assessed. This data
should be evaluated not only in the aggregate but also according to physician, age groups of physicians, location of practice, and share of surgery
procedures conducted at the respective hospitals. Only in this way can
the organization consider depth of demand by respective segments. The
analysis might reveal, for example, that the bulk of surgery is being conducted by a group of surgeons near retirement age. Thus, development of
a new ambulatory surgery center should be designed to attract new physicians.

Figure 2–4 Demand Analysis Sequence

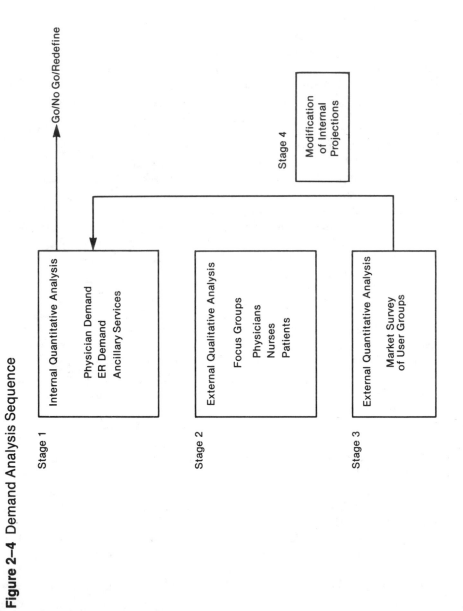

Similar internal analysis could be conducted for emergency department use according to service population base and the like. A particular concern in establishing ambulatory care services, such as primary care programs, is the extent to which additional revenue will be obtained from more patients, rather than just existing patients shifted from the emergency department to the primary care department.

Stage 2

If the internal analysis looks promising, the qualitative stage then would be conducted. At this point, focus group discussions would be conducted among prospective users of the proposed facility. Examples of focus groups have been provided elsewhere,[15,16] but generally these activities attempt to elicit emotional and subjective statements revealing the participants' preferences regarding the issues under discussion.

A focus group could be conducted with ten to twelve staff physicians whom the internal quantitative analysis revealed as likely users of the proposed surgery center. Discussions should focus on their existing perceptions of how such a facility operates; their experiences at different hospitals regarding surgical procedures; and the preferences for a more improved offered product. At the end of the discussion, the moderator of the focus group could describe the proposed facility and obtain reactions. Such a procedure might have revealed the travel problem between buildings described earlier.

Similarly, a focus group among consumers may help to clarify their perception of the offered product. Exhibit 2–1 contains sample focusing questions that could be used in such a session. Participants could be selected from the population at large and prescreened on prior surgery

---

Exhibit 2-1 Possible Focusing Questions for Prospective Patients

1. During your most recent hospital stay for surgery, what factors did you consider in determining the quality of care that was provided to you?
2. Many people say that some hospitals are better than others. In thinking about the last time you were in a hospital, what factors did you consider in deciding whether the hospital was good or bad?
3. In many places around the county, surgery is being conducted on an ambulatory basis—that is, people have surgery in the morning and are released at the end of the day. How do you think this procedure would work in this city?
4. What type of surgical procedures do you think most people would feel comfortable receiving in the type of facility just described? What do you think people would be concerned about?

experience. Suppose the questions are presented to participants in an area with no existing ambulatory surgery center. In this situation, the concept of not staying in the hospital after surgery may be more upsetting to a patient because of its novelty. This finding would indicate a need for a strong educational program. In areas where facilities do exist, community perceptions of them could be assessed.

The value of the focus group relates to Figure 2–3. The challenge for the hospital is to identify the generic components of the service. The qualitative stage must focus on understanding these components for each market. Generic components for consumers will differ from those for physicians.

A few guidelines should be followed in conducting this stage of research. Individuals involved in each focus group should be as homogeneous as possible. For example, all physicians should be from similar speciality areas; all consumers should be adults who have had surgery or should be parents of children who have had surgery. Unless all participants in the focus group can relate to the issue under discussion, the effectiveness of these sessions diminishes. Secondly, group moderators should be familiar with the problem under investigation so that they can probe for clarification of important issues. Finally, regardless of who conducts the focus group, data from these sessions should be analyzed by an individual outside the organization. One factor that becomes readily apparent is the subjective nature of focus groups. As a result, it becomes easy to interpret the data in whatever manner one desires. An independent judge can enhance the objectivity of the process. Although subjective in nature, this approach has been shown to have reasonable validity in examining research issues if conducted properly.[17]

Stage 3

The third stage entails an external quantitative assessment of demand. At this stage, the interest and perceptions of respective users, such as physicians, can be assessed on a broader scale. A market survey should be conducted to examine the intention to use such a facility. This process requires a fairly detailed description of the proposed program. Only with a reasonably refined concept can the respondents provide reasonable answers. Surveys should be conducted among the several markets involved in using or providing the service.

Data from the external assessment should be analyzed from a market segmentation perspective. That is, it is unlikely that the ambulatory surgery proposal will be equally desirable to all surveyed. The task for the analyst is to develop a profile of the segment which expresses the greatest likelihood to "buy" the service.

A mail survey, for example, conducted in the patient service area for a hospital would evaluate the importance to the consumer of the generic components identified in the focus group. In addition, the research would assess the desirability of an alternative surgery program, such as a one-day surgery service. Analysis of the data could be conducted according to occupation. The attractiveness of a surgery program may differ, for example, between union and nonunion positions, the difference being based on health benefits and sick-day allowances. Regardless of the reasons for differences in desirability, the analyst's objective must be to profile the group most willing to use the service.

This segment analysis can profile the likely users. The organization must then determine: (1) whether the size of this group is worthwhile attracting, and (2) whether the level of service desired can be delivered.

Stage 4

Results of stage 4 lead to the fourth step of modifying the internal quantitative assessment and the "go/no/go/redefine" strategy shown in Figure 2–4. A redefinition strategy may be necessary if negative feelings to the proposed surgery center are received during stage 3. Redefinition should focus on the offered product in light of market responses. If variations on the service are significant, the organization may have to reenter the research process. Market reactions should be monitored continually as the service approaches operationalization. If this process is followed, Table 2–1 shows the cycle. On completion of the research and development of the program in light of market responses, the hospital does not have to sell the program to physicians or consumers but rather inform these groups that the desired program is available.

The development of ambulatory surgery centers from a marketing perspective requires several prior considerations. The organization that recognizes the existence of multiple publics, with differing definitions for the service, is most likely to create a generic and offered product that appeals to the important user groups. Further, moreover, the demand analysis procedure should include a qualitative stage to test the concept and a quantitative analysis to estimate specific levels of interest in the area. The time required to conduct a detailed demand analysis may seem lengthy, but the cost of a wrong decision cannot be borne by any health provider in the present economic, regulatory, and competitive environment.

REFERENCES

1. Natof HE: Outpatient surgery: An alternative. *AORN Journal* 1979;29 (March):659–662.

2. MacStravic RE: Marketing health care services: The challenge of primary care. *Health Care Management Review* 1977;2 :9–15.

3. Drucker PF: *Management: Tasks, Responsibilities, Practices.* New York, Harper & Row Publishers, Inc, 1973, p 64.

4. Robeson FE: Health costs: Savings in the private sector. *California Management Review* 1979;21 (1979):49–56.

5. Grossman RE: Is ambulatory surgery less expensive? *Hospitals* 1979;53 (May):116.

6. *Federal Trade Commission News Summary,* Clanton outlines FTC budget proposals to house appropriations subcommittee. March 20, 1981.

7. Knauer V: Health care delivery in the future: The consumer's perspective. Read before the Learning Resource Center, St. Louis University Medical Center, St. Louis, MO, October 1979.

8. Kotler P: Strategies for introducing marketing into nonprofit organizations. *Journal of Marketing* 1979;43 (January):40.

9. Christianson JB, McClure W: Competition in the delivery of medical care. *Eng Med* 1979;301 (October):812–818.

10. Chase RB: Where does the customer fit in a service operation? *Harvard Business Review* 1978;56 (November–December):137–142.

11. Berry LL: Services marketing is different. *Business* 1980;30 (May–June):25–26.

12. Kovner AR, Smits HL: Consumer expectations of ambulatory care. *Health Care Management Review* 1978;3:69–75.

13. Lachner BJ: Marketing—An emerging management challenge. *Health Care Management Review* 1977;2:27.

14. Levitt T: Marketing success through differentiation of anything. *Harvard Business Review* 1980;58 (January–February): 83.

15. Flexner, WA, Berkowitz EN: Marketing research in health services planning: A model. *Public Health Reports* 1979:94 (November–December):503–513.

16. Flexner, WA, McClaughlin CP, Littlefield JE: Discovering what the health consumer wants. *Health Care Management Review* 1979:2:43–49.

17. Reynolds FD, Johnson DK: Validity of focus group findings. *Journal of Advertising Research* 1978;18 (June):21–24.

Chapter 3

Developing the Ambulatory Surgical Unit: The Physician's Responsibility

James E. Davis, M.D.

The development of ambulatory surgery has depended on the interest, participation, and leadership provided by physicians. The first authenticated report of operative surgery under general anesthesia with same-day discharge of the patient was made by a physician, James H. Nicoll, who in 1909 reported a large series of operative cases performed at the Glasgow Royal Hospital for Sick Children from 1899 to 1908. The first report of American participation in this form of surgical care came in September 1918, when R.W. Waters, M.D., of Sioux City, Iowa, reported similar cases at his Downtown Anesthesia Clinic. That such surgery was later being done in greater volume, at a limited number of sites, is emphasized by the report of Gertrude Hersfeld, M.D., in 1938, of a thousand hernia operations performed at the Royal Edinburgh Hospital for Sick Children.

The first modern program of such outpatient surgery in the United States, and the first in this country to be hospital sponsored and hospital based, was instituted at the University of California at Los Angeles Center for Health Sciences in 1962 by two anesthesiologists, David D. Cohen, M.D., and John B. Dillon, M.D.

In 1970 two other anesthesiologists, Wallace Reed, M.D., and John Ford, M.D., established the now noted Surgicenter® in Phoenix; many institutions, both hospital sponsored and freestanding independent, subsequently began to operate in the United States, almost invariably due to the initiative and leadership by physicians.

Now that ambulatory surgery is an established, well-developed, and fully accepted method of delivering surgical care, physicians must continue to play a vital role in the extension and greater availability of this safe, convenient, and cost-effective mode of care. More new ambulatory surgical units, enlarged and more efficient existing units, and units with greater

Adapted from *Journal of Ambulatory Care Management* 1981;3:27–34.

accessibility are needed. Physicians, especially surgeons, must see that these ends are accomplished. In the organization and planning of such units, the physicians' leadership is essential, and their responsibility is clearly mandated.

As vital as physician participation and direction are in the planning of a program of ambulatory surgery, physicians alone, with only minimal support and help from other hospital personnel, and without broad-based surgical, nursing, administrative, and trustee support cannot produce effective planning. It is necessary for representatives of all branches of the institution to participate with enthusiasm and conviction. True team effort is absolutely essential.

BASIC REQUIREMENTS

Those most interested in developing a modern ambulatory surgical unit must ensure that their institution and the leaders assembled for this purpose fulfill three requirements.

1. They must be aware of the capabilities of such units; the cost in time, effort, and dollars; the essentialness of meticulous planning; the trained personnel required in the planning and operation of such a unit; resultant changes in the institution's mix of surgical inpatients; and changes in practice and referral patterns in the community.

2. They must convince themselves that a sincere desire exists on the part of the institution and its leaders to have such a unit—a desire based on conviction that the unit will truly benefit the institution, the medical staff, the patients who use the institution, and the community.

3. The group must determine that a need exists, in the institution and throughout the referral community, for such a unit. Often the need for a unit is thought to be equated with the need for more surgical beds. This assumption is not necessarily the case, nor should it be.

When an adequate number of surgical beds are available, it would be more economical and allow more appropriate patient care if some beds were used for ambulatory surgical purposes. The institution with an excess of surgical beds is advised not to ignore the benefits of ambulatory surgery. It should consider either converting some beds to less costly ambulatory beds and converting other excess space to different revenue producing services, or using such unneeded space, at much less basic maintenance cost, for nonpatient purposes.

PLANNING TEAM

Once the decision to proceed has been made, the importance of team effort must be reemphasized to all participants, and representatives of this team must come from every segment of the institution. Specifically they should be members of the medical staff, representatives of nursing services, spokespeople for the administration, trustees of the institution, and members of the body that has ultimate responsibility for the institution (when this differs from the board of trustees).

Medical Staff

From the medical staff there must be representatives of multiple surgical divisions. One or even a few of the surgical divisions cannot successfully undertake such a project, and ideally all divisions of surgical care should be involved. Anesthesiologists not only are important to the planning and functioning of an ambulatory surgical unit, they are critical to its success and must participate early in the planning process.

Because the work of this unit will involve those outside the surgical-anesthesia areas, the chairperson of the department of radiology and the chairperson of the department of laboratories also should be invited to participate. Frequently surgeons who may not have leadership roles or administrative responsibilities within the hospital but are individually interested in this concept make valuable members of the team. Certainly the officers and leaders of the medical staff, insofar as they are not already representing the departments of surgery or anesthesiology, must actively participate in this work from the beginning.

Nursing Services

Nursing services also should be deeply involved in this new project, not only because nursing care is intrinsic to the unit but also because of the impact of the unit and its patients on nursing services throughout the hospital. Consequently, the director of nursing services must be fully informed of all planning and ideally will participate in the planning process. The supervisor of the operating suite and the nurse director of ambulatory services are also essential nursing representatives. Often individual nurses—especially those with a background relating to the operating suite, recovery rooms, or intensive care units—will become interested in this project, usually because of a desire to work in such a unit. These nurses also can become valuable members of the team.

Administration and Governing Body

From the administrative staff of the hospital, the chief executive officer and the senior administrator for ambulatory services are essential members of the team, as are the chief engineer, the comptroller, the chief reimbursement officer, the director of admitting services, and the public information officer. Their administrative areas will be involved in the proper functioning of such a new unit, and the early involvement of these leaders is necessary.

The board of trustees must be involved throughout the planning process, and their representatives should be participants on the planning team. Specifically the chairperson of the board, or his or her designee, and the chairperson of such pertinent committees as the committee on planning, the committee on finance, and the committee on buildings and grounds should be working members of the planning team. Not only will they make valuable contributions to the planning effort, but they can later help to obtain approval of final plans from the board of trustees.

If the governing authority of the hospital lies outside the board of trustees, representatives of this ultimate governing board also should be conversant with these matters and should be given the opportunity to contribute to the plan. If the institution is under local governmental control, representatives from the city council or the county commissioner's office would be appropriate. If the institution is church-related, clerical authorities should be invited. In the university setting, trustees of the university also should be knowledgeable about the accomplishments of this group. In the private corporate setting, representatives of the board should be involved.

STEERING COMMITTEE

The team as outlined has representatives from all the essential elements of the "hospital family," but its size has probably reduced its efficiency. Consequently, a steering committee of the group is likely to function more effectively. This committee should be small but should include one or more representatives from the department of surgery, the department of anesthesiology, the nursing services (particularly the division of ambulatory services), hospital administration, and the comptroller's (chief finance officer's) office. This smaller group then must fulfill, in sequence, specific functions.

The steering committee must *become fully informed* about what ambulatory surgical units are accomplishing in the early 1980s, and must be able to plan for reasonable expansion and improvement of services in the foreseeable future. This task can be accomplished by a thorough review of the literature, which can be done by one of more members of the committee, with the help of the librarian. An executive summary then can be prepared for other members.

Committee members also can become more informed by attending regional and national seminars that specifically address ambulatory surgery. The American Hospital Association, Division of Ambulatory Care, presents such programs periodically. Local and regional agencies such as Blue Cross and Blue Shield Associations and chapters of the American College of Surgeons offer similar information and guidance that addresses a specific unit's particular problems.

It is an excellent idea for members of the steering committee to *visit functioning units* to fully understand how they operate. This observation will help the committee better visualize what they want their units to become.

With this background information in hand, fully discussed and understood, the steering committee must begin to *make specific space and structural decisions* as to the design of the unit, the number of operating rooms, the square footage of each component of the unit, and the flow of traffic through the unit.

OPERATIONAL DECISIONS

At this stage, the steering committee also must *make operational decisions* that are contingent on further refinement and approval by the parent committee and ultimate authorities; however, these latter groups will need specific recommendations to which they can react. Specific categories of operational decisions are jurisdiction; director; privileges; patient selection; scheduling, charges, and payment policies; days and hours of operation; hospital admission; staffing; medical records; required laboratory procedures, and patient follow-up.

1. Administratively, will this unit, when established, be autonomous and self-contained, an extension of the operating room, or under the jurisdiction of ambulatory services?
2. The unit should have one individual who serves as director with the ultimate responsibility for the standards and quality of care, proper staffing, and maintenance of the physical plant. A second individual should be authorized to make decisions concerning the unit. In most instances, the individual should be a physician. The reporting responsibilities of this physician (directly to the hospital administrator, to the chairperson of the department of surgery, to the medical council, etc.) should be determined.
3. Who is going to use this unit? Members of the institution's surgical staff who are already privileged to use the operating rooms? All members of the community who are properly credentialed by a

hospital in the community? If endoscopic and other diagnostic or noncutting procedures are to be allowed, what is the status of non-surgeons who perform these procedures but are not privileged to use the institution's operating rooms?

4. Should a list be prepared of procedures that will be allowed in the unit, or is this decision to be left to the discretion of the licensed and board-certified physicians who use the unit?

5. The procedures for admitting patients to the unit and for scheduling operations must be determined. Will these tasks be done within the unit or will the hospital's admitting office arrange for admissions and schedule operating suite personnel for the ambulatory procedure? What are reasonable and equitable charges? Will there be an all-inclusive fee for a procedure, or will it be based on time plus charges for specific supplies and equipment? Because these procedures will be nonemergent, will financial responsibility for the charges have to be established before the patient enters the unit? Approval for this type of surgery must be solicited from all insurers in the area.

6. Which days of the week will the unit operate and during which hours?

7. Specific arrangements must be made for admission to the hospital of those few patients who are not ready to return home at the closing time of the unit. Such admissions usually result because of surgery being extended beyond anticipated limits, undue pain, or excess bleeding.

8. Will the staffing be autonomous to the unit or will there be personnel rotated from the operating rooms, recovery rooms, and department of anesthesia? How many individuals at each level of training and competence will be needed to care for patients undergoing surgery of this magnitude?

9. Will special records be prepared for use in the unit or will standard hospital forms be used? Will the short-form history, physical examination, and abbreviated discharge summary be sufficient? Specific standards and rules as to record keeping must be adopted.

10. Will specific requirements such as chest film, complete blood count, and urinalysis be required of all patients, and additionally an electrocardiogram required of patients over forty years of age? Or will the procedures ordered be left to the surgeon's judgment in each case, except for the simple hematocrit and "dip-stick" urinalysis required by the Joint Commission on Accreditation of Hospitals (JCAH) in such units?

11. Will patients be telephoned on the first postoperative day with an inquiry about their well-being and an evaluation of level of recovery? Will questionnaires be sent to patients (or to their surgeons) with the request that they be returned? Will return visits to the unit be allowed for changing of dressings or removal of sutures?

The steering committee, having come to an agreement on its recommendations concerning the preceding considerations, is prepared to formulate a general plan for the construction and operation of the unit. The entire planning team is then called back into session, and the steering committee's recommendations are presented for review. At this time, if not given previously, architectual advice is necessary so that the parent committee can make specific recommendations. These recommendations will be incorporated and accepted as the improved plan to be presented to the decision makers for their consideration and ultimate acceptance.

IMPLEMENTATION

With the final plan adopted and the project approved by the various bodies whose concurrence is essential, construction can get underway. During this phase, much can be done to inform and educate the profession, the public, and the media about the advantages of ambulatory surgery.

Education

A formal series of educational programs concerning the purpose, the function, and the anticipated accomplishments of the unit should be presented as effectively as possible and should first address the entire medical staff. Even those members of the medical staff who will not be using the unit should fully understand its function and the low-risk factor involved. Many of them will have occasion to refer patients for this type of care, and their opinion, understanding, and enthusiasm for ambulatory surgery will greatly influence their patients' decision to accept it. Subsequently, the entire referring medical community should be briefed on this type of care and encouraged to recommend it to their patients.

As construction continues and the actual date of opening is anticipated, all hospital personnel should be thoroughly instructed and informed about the new unit; the office personnel of all members of the medical staff also should be invited to the hospital to learn about the new (to community) and innovative method of providing surgical care. The news media should be extensively briefed so that they can help to educate the public about this type of operative care.

Preopening Activities

The preopening activities should be carefully planned and executed. Publicity concerning the unit should be increased, and informational brochures for patients and potential patients should be prepared and made available throughout the hospital and in the office of every member of the medical staff. Open-house visitations should be arranged for the medical community, the trustees and governing bodies, the hospital employees, the physicians' office personnel, and the news media so that everyone can be given the opportunity to see the impressive facilities for themselves.

VALUE

The planning process, long and at times arduous, has been completed; the unit is functioning; and physician leadership and contributions have been evident and needed at every step. The question arises, even among the hardiest, Has it been worth it? To those who have been through it, the answer inevitably is yes!

In the 1980s the unnecessary use of inpatient beds, unjustified additional costs, and the unwarranted high level of care that results from hospitalizing patients who have a low level of surgical need cannot be condoned. It is highly satisfying to have these patients adequately and appropriately cared for in the ambulatory unit and to save dollars, beds, and time without sacrificing the quality of care. Physicians should realize that this is not only cost-effective medicine but good medicine.

Chapter 4

Ambulatory Surgery: A Surgeon's Point of View

Richard O. Kraft, M.D., F.A.C.S.

GENERAL DISCUSSION

History

Surgical practice during the first half of the twentieth century was characterized by expertise in minor procedures to an extent almost forgotten by those of more recent training. Christopher and others published excellent textbooks that gave detailed descriptions of techniques suitable for the office in the management of a variety of acquired abnormalities, congenital defects, and injuries.[1] The explosion of hospital construction following World War II and the tendency of highly specialized practices to focus on inpatient care led to a decline in outpatient procedure activity. The current wave of enthusiasm for this mode of care dates from the experiences published by the faculty of the University of California at Los Angeles,[2] Hill on the East Coast,[3] and the development of the world famous Surgicenter® in Phoenix, Arizona, by Ford and Reed.[4]

The present momentum is away from standard-term inpatient surgical care and toward short-stay, ultra-short-stay (including preadmit testing and twenty-three-hour bed occupancy), and ambulatory surgery. This shift has occurred despite an excess of hospital beds, an abundance of operating room capacity, and a progressive increase in acuity of care. Public and professional awareness as to costs of health care are in part responsible for this improvement, and insurance companies similarly have been vocal in encouragement. Ambulatory surgery presents the ultimate in cost saving as regards the "hotel component" of surgical expense. There is a considerable evidence of progressive acceptance of this technique. One regional study indicates an improvement in usage from less than 8 percent to over 25 percent in an eight-year period.[5] The spectacular growth of independent ambulatory surgery units throughout the past decade is additive to hospital-sponsored program development.

Safety

Patient safety is the paramount concern of all health providers. It is clear that ambulatory surgery in a properly organized and staffed facility is a safe method of care. The Freestanding Ambulatory Surgical Association has compiled an extraordinary report of over seventy thousand operations performed in 1980 with no deaths, a single transfusion required, and 0.3 percent frequency of transfer necessitated to inpatient status; only eight of the 223 transfers were considered emergent.[6] Postoperative infections have actually been found to be less frequent.[7] The author's experience with ambulatory surgery utilizing inpatient hospital operating rooms confirms an admission rate of 2 percent. In such circumstances, a more cavalier attitude toward an overnight stay would be expected, as would a tendency perhaps to undertake more extensive procedures as contrasted to freestanding, independent, and isolated units. These records represent ambulatory surgery performed in exemplary style. They have been accumulated from facilities fulfilling the requirements for certification by accrediting bodies. Careful patient selection and preoperative evaluation are required for such certification, and quality assurance measures also are critically reviewed.

Anesthesia

The increasing interest in ambulatory surgery has been a product of developments in surgical techniques and philosophy, patients' acceptance, and cost awareness. None of these factors, however, have been nearly as influential as the revolution in anesthesiology. Physicians in this specialty have enjoyed rapidly expanding interest and responsibility in intensive care, prolonged respiratory support, pain control, operating room administration, and innovative developments such as ambulatory care programs. Exciting new technical and pharmacological developments have occurred simultaneously, including ultra-short-acting anesthetic agents and modified techniques in conduction anesthesia. The expansion of ambulatory surgery owes more to the field of anesthesiology than any other single factor.

Economics

In the past, the patient and physician represented a "cost-conscious consumer partnership." Each partner shared in the savings achieved in the management of illness. The surgeon providing office care at twenty dollars was popular; less so was the surgeon insisting on expensive hospitalization for a similar illness. Now U.S. citizens enjoy almost universal medical insurance (though of varying quality), minimizing this cost consciousness. Although most insurance policies provide for professional surgical fees regardless of the setting in which procedures are performed, few offer facility reimbursement (for costs related to consumables, sterilization and processing, and nursing assistants) for procedures performed in the physician's office. Such facility costs in hospital settings are routinely covered. The effect is to shift technical procedures from the more economical office to the more expensive hospital inpatient service. Consequently, even large modern group-practice offices rarely have minor operating rooms. Plastic surgeons, in contrast, almost always have well-equipped office surgeries, since approximately 50 percent of their practices are "self-pay" cosmetic operations.

New developments in health service financing may alter the relationship between surgeon's offices, ambulatory surgery facilities, and traditional inpatient surgical activities. The national Blue Cross and Blue Shield Associations are experimenting with "facility fee adjustments" for minor procedures performed in surgeon's offices. Health maintenance organizations will focus attention on cost containment methods that will increase the use of office techniques as well as ambulatory facilities. Government health insurance plans (Medicaid and Medicare) are at this time introducing *mandated* lists of operations to be performed in an outpatient mode only, at the risk of reduced reimbursement. The complexities of hospital accounting practices coupled with prospective reimbursement (in some regions) also provide strong encouragement for shifts to the ambulatory setting.

MAKING THE DECISION

The Physician and the Patient

Patients undergoing surgery in the ambulatory mode are universally satisfied, or at least are more satisfied than patients undergoing comparable procedures on an inpatient basis. Lessened family disruption and inconvenience, and the comfort and reassurance of one's home surroundings are contributing factors. The surgeon, however, basically controls the gate and method for delivery of surgical care. It is encouraging then to read reports of consistent (over 90 percent) satisfaction from the practitioner's perspective as well. This positive attitude is related to efficiency in time and procedure performance. The ambulatory mode eliminates the need for preoperative and postoperative inhospital patient-physician contact; enables operating rooms to minimize "down time" between cases; and facilitates "block scheduling," which further benefits the surgeon. Cancellations and shifts in timing are rare in the ambulatory setting since only elective operations are permitted, and accurate time estimates are characteristics of these commonly performed brief procedures. Surgeons practicing in specialities characterized by large numbers of quick, purely elective operations (e.g., ear, nose, throat, plastic surgery, eye) are particularly pleased with the arrangements offered.

Patients and surgeons alike share some concerns regarding in-and-out surgery, not the least of which has to do with tradition. There is a need for both physician and patient education, because change always arouses anxiety and reluctance. More effort is required of the surgeon's office personnel; patients should receive explicit preparation, instruction, and coordination rather than simply being instructed to report to the admitting desk. Patient compliance with instructions is suspect, though rarely a significant problem on analysis. In comparing outpatients with inpatients, intercurrent illness occurs no more and perhaps less frequently among patients with comparable surgical problems. Specific attention must be focused on the preoperative laboratory, x-ray and cardiographic studies, the history and physical reports, and the operative permit. The surgeon's office staff must be compulsive; their responsibility is to have all this material at the center forty-eight hours prior to the operative day. This facet is the single most troublesome area in the entire process.

Those surgeons already performing a significant volume of ambulatory surgery are easily encouraged to expand this mode of care when a new program is initiated or an old program improved. Hospital staffs with a high percentage of cardiac surgeons and neurosurgeons are likely to be less enthusiastic about ambulatory surgery programs than staffs in hospitals with large numbers of gynecologists, otorhinolaryngologists, and plastic surgeons. The development of an ambulatory surgery program may purposely encourage the development of a more rounded and balanced staff.

The physician's age has been demonstrated to be a factor in accepting innovative concepts of care. Younger physicians in general are most adaptable. This principle has been demonstrated at St. Joseph Mercy Hospital in Ann Arbor, Michigan, where the success of efforts made to shorten the average length of stay (because of high bed occupancy) was inversely proportional to the age of the surgeons (see Table 4–1).

Hospitals with postgraduate educational responsibilities find themselves in somewhat of a dilemma. It is difficult for house officers to see the patients preoperatively as well as postoperatively when the surgical pro-

Table 4-1 Influence of Surgeon's Age and Education Effort on Average Length of Stay (ALOS) of Adult Inguinal Herniorrhaphies

ALOS (Days)*		Number of Operations	Number of Surgeons	Surgeon's Average Age
1972	5.5	322		
	>6.0(7.4)	50	4	50
	<4.5(4.1)	53	3	43
1976	4.0	233		
	>5.0(5.7)	35	5	54
	<3.0(2.4)	23	2	48

Source: St. Joseph Mercy Hospital.

*The ALOS in 1977 was 5.3.

cedure is performed in the ambulatory facility. Review committees in surgery recognize this modern form of care, however, and now require some outpatient experience as part of the training of every doctor. Surgical specialists in teaching hospitals have long enjoyed the privilege of having the history and physical, provided by the house officer, the night before the operation. Innovative scheduling, the use of physician's extenders, and the preanesthesia facility visit all may serve to overcome this hurdle. An extra, preoperative day of hospitalization for this sole purpose, however, is not acceptable.

A regional analysis also must be undertaken in measuring patient satisfaction and preferences. Population growth expectations alone will not suffice. Distances traveled are important, with thirty miles considered the upper limit of acceptability. St. Joseph Mercy Hospital's studies have indicated an inverse ratio between patient satisfaction and geographic dislocation. This factor is relative to patient safety as well. These programs are particularly adaptable to young adults and children. Students, however, frequently live alone in small apartments and are unlikely candidates. Hospitals in small communities with far-reaching tertiary care referral patterns are ill-suited for heavy investment in ambulatory surgery programs. Initiating such a program in a tertiary facility may be appropriate, however, for purposes of broadening the spectrum of care and diminishing financial problems related to high-acuity patient population.

The total regional analysis must include the population served, the characteristics of that population, the number of operating rooms available, the number of operations performed, the ratio of ambulatory surgery currently performed to total operations performed, and the percentage of bed occupancy.

A general formula for regional analysis would include as favorable characteristics:

1. A high-density, youthful, and expanding population base.
2. Large hospitals with high occupancy and high operating room rates.
3. A young and dynamic medical staff.
4. Responsive third party payers.

Useful norms would include:

1. One thousand inpatient operations per operating room per year.
2. Bed occupancy of 85 percent.
3. Outpatient surgeries ranging from 25 to 40 percent of total surgeries (target).
4. Fifteen hundred operations per operating room per year (ambulatory surgery program target).
5. Greater than two thousand operations per year per outpatient program or facility (target).

Impact on Regional Hospitals

High fixed costs and complex methods of compensation and allocation leave hospitals susceptible to variations in patient days and shifts in the spectrum of complexity of care. The hospital least affected by a new ambulatory surgery program in its region is one that owns and manages the unit while experiencing high demand for all services. Hospitals with low occupany and excess surgical resources face a serious challenge.[5] These hospitals should consider ambulatory surgery programs even in the face of low occupancy since such programs (1) attract physicians and their patients to the facility, and (2) decrease the acuity-of-care factor. Such a hospital may temporarily or permanently need to close beds or shift to innovative alternate care concepts for these beds (e.g., rehabilitation, substance abuse, skilled nursing extended care, etc.).

Types of Programs

Small ambulatory surgery programs (less than two thousand cases per year) may best be incorporated into the main hospital facility. This "day-surgery" methodology works quite well for small numbers of patients and is the least expensive way to provide this mode of care. Smaller hospitals,

with their generally lower occupancy rates and less efficient use of operating rooms, are particularly appropriate for this system. Small hospitals
also tend to be rural and are therefore less likely to have successful major
programs in ambulatory surgery.

Large hospitals with high bed occupancy and heavy use of operating
rooms should strongly consider an ambulatory surgery facility on campus—ideally with an all-weather connecting link. An isolated unit in the
main building serves equally well in the unlikely circumstance of available
space. The separation of inpatients and outpatients is extremely important
to the function of such programs. The outpatient "second-class citizen"
status thus is obviated. Personnel morale and program efficiency benefit.
Location on campus increases program efficiency by permitting the sharing
of basic services (security, maintenance, heat, laundry), and emergency
support is at hand in the rare instances it is required. In addition, the
campus location permits a (limited) expansion of the spectrum of cases
performed in contrast to isolated facilities. Physician convenience is a
strong marketing factor.

Independent, freestanding units are highly efficient. They have been
well received by surgeons and patients alike. The data available indicates
high professional standards, and an enviable safety record. Unit costs are
lower than those achieved by comparable hospital-related programs. The
greatest difficulties experienced by such facilities have been those of approval
through the certificate-of-need process and recognition by third party
payers. Each year, more insurance companies recognize these facilities
for reimbursement. Regional health authorities question potential conflict
of interest, and possible increase in total regional surgical rates. Hospital
influences on the political process may constitute a significant resistance
factor as well.

MEDICAL CONSIDERATIONS

Expectations

The federal government has suggested that 25 percent of all surgeries
be performed on an ambulatory basis. Phoenix, Arizona, demonstrated an
increase from 5 percent to 30 percent in less than a decade.[5] Burns and
Ferber[8] report that 16.4 percent of the surgical operations in U.S. hospitals
are currently being performed on an outpatient basis. Hertzler (personal
communications, 1981) indicates that Children's Hospital in Detroit is now
at 40 percent. St. Joseph Mercy Hospital has increased the percentage of
ambulatory surgery from 13 percent in 1971 to 27 percent in 1980 (3,897

outpatient procedures; 14,535 total operations). This figure excludes 1,964 endoscopies, 545 outpatient cystoscopies, and 214 office procedures. The 25 percent national guideline is an appropriate figure. Thirteen of the twenty-five most common operations performed in the United States are appropriate for ambulatory management (see Table 4–2).[9]

Selling the Program

Traditional concerns are lessened through continuing educational efforts. Surgeons now recognize that problems directly related to wounds generally are not related to hospital confinement or to activity. Mild hematoma formation rarely is of significance, and if bleeding becomes a major problem, it is almost always recognized while the patient is in the postanesthesia recovery unit. Wound tensile strength is greater during the first forty-eight hours following the operation than during the following week—a fact that negates the importance of a brief hospitalization for "protection" from disruption. Wound infections may actually be less frequent in the ambulatory setting.[7] A careful review of the author's experience regarding inpatient surgery indicates that wound infections are more apt to occur during the second postoperative week than during the first seven days.[10] Modern concepts minimize the historic attention paid to postoperative

---

Table 4-2 Operations Suitable for Outpatient Surgery—Thirteen of the Twenty-five Most Common Operations

Rank	Operation	ALOS	Applicability†
1	Dilatation and curettage	2.7	**
3	Hernia	5.6	*
5	Tonsillectomy and adenoidectomy	1.9	***
7	Cystoscopy	6.6	*
8	Cataract	4.9	**
9	Breast biopsy	3.7	***
10	Skin suture	8.3	*
14	Skin lesion	5.1	*
15	Esophogastroscopy	9.3	?
16	Tonsil	2.3	***
18	Myringotomy tube placement	2.1	***
20	Tooth extraction	3.1	***
21	Cardiac catheterization	5.7	*

Source: St. Joseph Mercy Hospital, 1977.

†Somewhat(*) to highly(***) applicable.

dressings, with some surgeons actually recommending bathing the first postoperative day.

The only modern development of concern is that of potential litigation—malpractice. Statistically, complex surgery carries a greater potential for adverse results, which in turn increases the potentiality of litigation. Elective procedures of modest extent almost always are followed by a favorable outcome. Careful documentation and accuracy of records, including informed consent, are strongly recommended. The nationwide acceptance of ambulatory surgery as a safe standard should ameliorate this concern.

"Preferential scheduling" has helped in accelerating the acceptance of ambulatory surgery at St. Joseph Mercy Hospital. Outpatient operating room time consistently is made more available than that scheduled for inpatients.

Specific Speciality Considerations

Certain speciality services predominate in ambulatory surgery facilities. Gynecology, otorhinolaryngology, and plastic surgery are particularly suited to such facilities; cardiothoracic surgery and neurosurgery rarely are performed. It is valuable to analyze current practices in identifying specialties that are active in the ambulatory surgery mode, those on which educational endeavor could be focused, and those that have particular problems requiring identification and correction.

Gynecology

This specialty predominates in essentially all ambulatory surgical units. Dilatation and curettage is the most common operation performed in the United States annually and is particularly suited to ambulatory surgery. A small percentage of these procedures are performed in offices under paracervical block anesthesia, but the usual pattern is that of inpatient care with an average length of stay of 2.6 days. The percentage of ambulatory care related to this particular operation has increased from zero to 65 percent at St. Joseph Mercy Hospital over the past ten years. Another procedure commonly performed in ambulatory surgery programs is laparoscopy. When laparotomy is anticipated, the main operating room is the appropriate setting (e.g., in the diagnosis of suspected ectopic pregnancy).

The outpatient system also is ideal for elective infertility examinations and tubal interruptions. Sterilizations usually represent 10 percent of the annual surgical volume in ambulatory programs. Pregnancy interruptions are rarely performed in general ambulatory surgical facilities. Cryosurgery and laser surgery progressively will influence the practices in this speciality as well as in others.

Otorhinolaryngology

The elective nature of patient care and the brief duration of the operative procedures, with subsequent prompt recovery, encourage block-scheduling techniques and are a factor in the popularity of day surgery with otorhinolaryngologists. Large segments of operating room time may be held available for those specialists who demonstrate consistent usage. Unscheduled residual time is given over to the general scheduling process in advance at an arbitrary time (e.g., one week). This method of scheduling provides the utmost in efficiency for the facility and the ultimate in satisfaction for the patient and surgeon. Tonsillectomies have been shown to be a safe procedure for the ambulatory mode, but some surgeons still express concern over delayed hemorrhage. Lieberman[11] reported that of four thousand outpatient tonsillectomies, only 1.5 percent required an overnight stay. Fully three quarters of the patients ultimately hospitalized were identified during their postanesthesia recovery; sixteen of the four thousand cases developed delayed complications. If accepted, tonsillectomies will prove to be a large-volume procedure. This operation may require specific surgeon-privilege review since wide variations in outcome seem characteristic. Modern ear, nose, and throat procedures do require microscopic instrumentation, which adds to the procedure cost and the complexity of minor scheduling (although the latter is obviated by block scheduling).

Urology

Many urologic procedures are appropriate for the ambulatory surgery facility but require special equipment to operate cystoscopes, irrigation systems, and tables. Block scheduling circumvents the problem of converting and reconverting a room for urologic procedures and other specialties. Tables are available that are readily altered and converted. Special attention must be paid to state public health stipulations to avoid the error of committing one operating room for a single specialty purpose. (This error should be avoided in any case because it impairs the efficiency of scheduling and usage.) Occasionally, endoscopic diagnostic procedures subtly become major therapeutic endeavors, which may exceed expectations. Specific monitoring of surgeons may be necessary. Some programs have avoided cystoscopic procedures for various reasons, but if permitted, these operations do become a significant numerical factor.

Plastic Surgery

Elective procedures of minimal risk are ideal for outpatient management. The self-pay characteristic of cosmetic surgery is further incentive to seek this cost-effective mode. Time estimates are sometimes faulty, but block scheduling is applicable. Microscopic procedures of this specialty tend to be lengthy, and may have to be excluded because of schedule overruns and slow postoperative recovery.

General Surgery

Pediatric procedures in general surgery as well as in the other surgical specialties have been particularly well received. The psychological impact on patient and family is minimized, and the chance of incurring hospital-related infection is lessened. Pediatric surgeons in particular are in uniform support of this mode of care. Herniorrhaphies in young patients, as well as in some adults, have been increasingly well received.

The two-stage approach to breast disease (i.e., a biopsy performed on an ambulatory basis, followed by definitive intervention, if necessary, at a later date) has been a tremendous advance. Eighty percent of breast biopsies are benign, and the outpatient procedure suffices. When the biopsy is positive for neoplasm, a delay of a week or two has no adverse impact and permits in-depth discussion and consultation so characteristic of this disease.[12] Rapid processing of the tissue should be available to enable appropriate special chemical determinations to be undertaken (e.g., estrogen receptor analysis). General surgeons use the ambulatory surgery facility only intermittently and tend, therefore, not to gain the benefits of block scheduling.

Orthopedic Surgery

Until recently the orthopedic surgeon has been an infrequent visitor to the ambulatory surgery facility. Appropriate operations included removal of pins and hardware along with carpal tunnel release and tendon transfers. Arthroscopy has changed the order of things. The equipment is expensive and requires special care and handling, often leading to the employment of an arthroscopy technician. This procedure will substitute for many open arthrotomies, which are associated with significant disability and inpatient requirements. Arthroscopy was the tenth most frequent outpatient procedure performed in 1980 (see Table 4–3).[6]

Table 4-3 Ten Most Common Operations, 1980

1. Dilatation and curettage
2. Myringotomy
3. Tubal ligation
4. Orthopedic procedures
5. Dental procedures
6. Excision of skin lesion
7. Diagnostic laparoscopy
8. Tonsillectomy and/or adenoidectomy
9. Cystoscopy
10. Arthroscopy

Source: Freestanding Ambulatory Surgical Association, 1980.

Ophthalmology

As in general surgery, ophthalmology patients ideally suited to the ambulatory surgery program are in the pediatric age group, which undergoes operations for muscle imbalance, examinations under anesthesia, and tear-duct probings. Cataract surgery has not been accepted universally as appropriate to the outpatient mode, but it has been performed extensively in some centers. Cataract extraction is the fourth most common outpatient procedure at St. Joseph Mercy Hospital.

Dental and Oral Surgery

Ambulatory care facilities offer expertise in anesthesia and postanesthesia recovery and are of tremendous value to specialists in dental and oral surgery. These professionals often find themselves dealing with major oral problems requiring greater support than is available in dental offices, but they are hampered by policy and traditional territorial constraints in the hospital setting.

Podiatry

Professional and government agencies are striving to delineate the health service spectrum position appropriate for podiatry. When the practice of podiatry is authorized in an ambulatory surgery program, it will constitute a major component of that program's activities.

Pain Control Clinics

A long-neglected area has been the control of chronic pain. Anesthesiologists recently have initiated great efforts in this direction, including such techniques as major nerve blocks and invasive testing. These activities are well suited to ambulatory surgery facilities. They are scheduled at the end of the day, since prompt recovery can be anticipated and the anesthesiologist is readily available.

Endoscopy

Esophagogastroscopy, colonoscopy, and bronchoscopy should be considered as a separate entity. These procedures rarely require general anesthesia, though a period of recovery from intravenous sedation is usual. When these procedures are carried out in an ambulatory surgery facility, the data base should indicate the fact to facilitate comparison analysis. The institutional assessment at St. Joseph Mercy Hospital has concluded that a separate endoscopy area in the main hospital is most appropriate, since 50 percent of these procedures are carried out on inpatients. Outpatients may be cared for within the inpatient setting, but state regulations prohibit the converse situation. Locating the center in single main hospital permits the performance of over two thousand such procedures annually while avoiding the duplication of facilities and staffing.

Minor Operation Room

A minor operation room, or "mini room," is an important part of an ambulatory surgery program. This small room is to be used by surgeons for limited procedures under local anesthesia with minimal assistance. This alternative eliminates the need to perform office procedures in the main operating room. A mini room also should be less expensive to use, should be responsive to flexible scheduling, and should require minimal paperwork (a log book and operative notes only). The nationwide popularity of these small rooms in ambulatory surgery facilities justifies their presence. Minor office procedures should be excluded from or so indicated in any data derived from ambulatory surgery facilities.

Lists of Operations

Insurance companies and government agencies repeatedly request lists of operations suitable for ambulatory surgery facilities. Clinicians caution against this practice, recognizing that such lists all too quickly become inclusive and exclusive. A refined list of suggested procedures,[13] under consideration by the Michigan Medicaid Planning Agency, includes twenty-six procedures, half of which are more suitable for office care than an ambulatory surgery facility. Some procedures, however, would be perfectly appropriate for inpatient scheduling under certain circumstances. There are simply too many variables involved to permit such simplification. External review for purposes of quality assurance or even regulation may better focus on institutional norms. The national target of having ambulatory procedures measuring 25 percent of the total operations performed may prove appropriate for standard acute-care general hospitals. Analyses of specific specialties will assist in identifying existing problems.

THE PROGRAM METHODOLOGY

Prefacility Phase

This phase is the most critical step in the program sequence. The key is an accurate preoperative, preanesthesia evaluation by the responsible surgeon or the surgeon's designee in collaboration and coordination with the anesthesiologist. The surgeon must recognize that the patient as well as the procedure must be appropriate to the ambulatory mode. The American Society of Anesthesiology accepts only risk-classes I and II patients (i.e., healthy patients or patients with well-controlled modest chronic abnormalities). Age is less a factor than physiological state. The patient and the family must be well informed and compliant. Distances involved must not be excessive, generally, twenty to thirty miles is considered a practical limit not only to facilitate patient comfort but also to assure the availability of the physician or surgeon should complications arise. Patients who live alone, are troubled by social or psychological disturbances, or have secondary but unstable physiological derangement should not be considered suitable.

The surgeon's responsibility is to obtain an accurate preanesthesia history and physical examination as well as information related to the chief complaint. Surgeons not qualified or unwilling to complete this preanesthesia evaluation must take alternate arrangements in conjunction with the responsible anesthesiologist. Such acceptable arrangements include completion of the appropriate evaluation by the family physician, acting as consultant, or a preanesthesia visit several days in advance with the anesthesiologist at the facility. Preanesthesia testing (laboratory, x-rays, cardiograms, etc.) are specifically dependent on the preanesthesia history and physical examination. Formulas based on age categories, though a poor compromise, are standard throughout the country. The author's review of cancellations of inpatient procedures revealed a 4 percent frequency rate, almost all unrelated to laboratory studies, electrocardiograms, and chest x-rays. No patient under the age of forty required cancellation on the basis of these ancillary studies. A change in the patient's general condition (i.e., intercurrent illness) was the most common problem (see Table 4–4).

Anesthesiologists have increasingly emphasized their willingness to participate in the preoperative evaluation. Approximately 50 percent of the ambulatory surgery programs require a preoperative visit several days before the procedure to serve this purpose. At the minimum, the anesthesiologist should have the privilege of reviewing all forms, laboratory data, and permits forty-eight hours prior to the procedure so that patients with possible complexities can be identified in advance and appropriate steps initiated on their behalf. Only in this way can safe care be provided and disruption of the schedule of the patient, surgeon, and facility be avoided. Nurse clinicians and physician's assistants will prove exceedingly helpful as will computer-assisted programs based on the patient's completed history and supplemental physical examinations. The preoperative visit should be made available to patients who desire it, and the preoperative evaluation should be made available to specialty surgeons who are having difficulty complying with the requirements. The surgeon also must directly or through the preanesthesia technique fully explain to the patients what is expected of them and what they in turn will experience preceding, during, and following the surgery.

Facility Phase

The patient should arrive sixty to ninety minutes prior to the scheduled operation. Preregistration should be complete and all paperwork finished.

Table 4-4 Surgery Cancellations

Elective cases reviewed	2,850
Change in condition	57
Nonmedical (e.g., patient refusal)	28
Surgeon related	15
Other	5
Preoperative testing not helpful	105
Preoperative testing helpful	16
EKG abnormal	8 (patient age 50–86 years)
Laboratory tests abnormal	7
Hb ↓	3 (48, 50, 80 years)
SGOT ↑	2 (60, 61 years)
K$^+$ ↓	1 (66 years)
WBC ↑ (2 yo, T°)	1 (0 years)
Chest x-ray abnormal	1 (87 years)
Cancellations	121 (4 percent)

Source: St. Joseph Mercy Hospital.

The time interval is important, however, in terms of correcting any deficits; confirming compliance with such requirements as "nothing by mouth," "no intercurrent illness," and "presence of escort" and identifying "no-show" patients early in the sequence.

The surgeon must be available prior to the induction of anesthesia so the patient and doctor can meet and discuss any remaining problems. If technical assistance is required for the operative procedure, the surgeon should make arrangements well in advance through either the facility services or other professionals. House officers are encouraged to participate, but the surgeon must remain in direct personal collaboration throughout the entire procedure in order to maintain the time efficiency so characteristic of successful ambulatory surgery programs.

The system should permit the completion of all forms prior to the patient's departure from the facility, including dictation of a formal operative note. Standard surgeon-specific or general-approved protocols for discharging patients from the facility are required, and must contain the phone number at which the surgeon can be reached if the patient experiences complexities at home.

The facility must be able to respond with both equipment and professional expertise to meet such extraordinary needs as blood transfusions, patient transfer, laparotomy for hemorrhage, and other intraoperative and perioperative problems. There is an inconsistent relationship between the duration of operation and the duration of recovery, but certain operations (e.g., laparoscopy) are associated with more than the usual discomfiture and delay in discharge. Additional future data of this type certainly will be of value.

Postfacility Phase

Prompt recovery is anticipated for properly selected patients and properly performed operations. Surgeons generally experience few postoperative calls, and these are rarely of significance. The time savings due to pre- and postoperative visits in the hospital more than compensate for the time taken to answer these calls. Certain operations seem to have specific characteristics; for example, adult patients undergoing outpatient inguinal herniorrhaphy under local anesthesia often demonstrate somewhat more edema and ecchymosis. None of these variations, however, appears to be significant.

Management

The management of ambulatory surgery programs should be as independent as is compatible with governance and ownership. The medical director carries the responsibility of patient management within the facility (i.e., the program) and must have authority appropriate to that responsibility. The right to cancel any case and to transfer any patient must reside with the medical director, who will, of course, consult with the appropriate responsible surgeon. The logical choice for medical director is an anesthesiologist with a particular interest in ambulatory surgery, although many programs have surgeons in this position. The medical director undoubtedly will share responsibilities with a head nurse or nurse-administrator and will require the assistance of a business manager in the performance of the many duties.

An advisory, or steering, committee serves an extremely important function. Representatives should include members from the departments and sections of surgery who use the program with high frequency. The purpose of the committee is to offer counsel and advice to the medical director and, in turn, to serve as a liaison with the surgeons on the staff.

Quality Assurance

Ambulatory surgery programs (i.e., the facilities) should request review and certification either by the Joint Commission on Accreditation of Hospitals (JCAH) or the Accreditation Association for Ambulatory Health Care (AAAHC). A standardized method for the analysis of end results should be characteristic of all ambulatory facilities; included in the analysis should be deaths, transfusions, transfers, infection rates, and cancellations. Data that is less explicit but of importance would include patient satisfaction, surgeon satisfaction, reasons for cancellations, and reasons for delays. Detailed studies that eventually will prove very helpful and that can be conducted with computer assistance are specific surgeon performance, measuring errors in time estimates, actual time required, and complication rates; and operation specifics, such as complication rates, time consumption, and special equipment used. To a great extent, success of the program depends on the efficiency of the system. Patient and surgeon satisfaction ultimately will be made clear by the numbers of visits processed in this new era of competitive health care delivery.

POTENTIAL HAZARDS

There is widespread concern over the movement toward open competition in an effort to control ever-accelerating health care costs. The seemingly endless demand by the population for health services seems to bear no relationship to health care need. There is consequently little hope that a balance of supply and demand will be achieved. Consumer fiscal responsibility would seem essential to the success of this new philosophy; yet copayment and less-than-total-care coverage meet with little political support. There is a potential risk of an overall increase in surgical costs in the future despite strong shifts to less expensive modes of care on a unit basis, such as ambulatory surgery. This adverse economic momentum would be compounded by a number of occurrences: a shift of office-level procedures to ambulatory surgery facilities; a decrease in bed occupancy on the inpatient side without the closing of beds and/or hospitals; and overconstruction of ambulatory surgery facilities, leading to a conflict of interest regarding conservation in the application of surgical care and fiscal responsibility between facility owners and creditors. The impending glut of physicians is of even greater significance. The Graduate Medical Education National Advisory Committee (GMENAC) report[14] is one of several studies projecting an astounding growth in physician manpower in the United States in the immediate future. Experience indicates that more physicians lead to more consumption of health services with increasing costs. A recent study confirms a 1 percent increase in total surgery rates when a 10 percent increase in numbers of surgeons per capita occurs.[15]

Ambulatory surgery is a safe alternative to inpatient care. More than 25 percent of all operations can be performed in this less expensive manner. Patients and surgeons are mutually supportive. The impact on total health care costs, however, has yet to be determined.

REFERENCES

1. Christopher F: *Minor Surgery*. Philadelphia, WB Saunders Co, 1929.

2. Cohen D, Dillon, JB: Anesthesia for outpatient surgery. *JAMA* 1966;196: 1114.

3. Hill : Outpatient surgery. *Hospital Administration Currents* 1972;16 (April): 1–4.

4. Ford J, Reed W: The Surgicenters®: An innovation in the delivery of medical care. *Arizona Medicine,* 1969;26 (October): 801–804.

5. Orkand D, Jaggar F, Hurwitz E: *Cooperative Evaluation of Costs, Quality, and System Effects of Ambulatory Surgery Performed in Alternate Alternative Settings.* US Dept of Health, Education, and Welfare, 1977.

6. Bruns K: Freestanding Ambulatory Surgery Association statistics in *Same-Day Surgery* 1981; (April): 47.

7. Lawrie R: Operating on children as day cases. *Lancet* 1964;2: 1289.

8. Burns L, Ferber M: Ambulatory surgery in the U.S.: Developments and prospects. *Journal of Ambulatory Care Management* 1981;3:1–13.

9. Commission on Professional and Hospital Activities: *Length of Stay in PAS Hospitals by Operation*. Ann Arbor, Mich, Commission on Professional and Hospital Activities, 1979.

10. Weber DO, Gooch JJ, Wood WR, et al: Influence of operating room surface contamination on surgical wounds. *Archives of Surgery* 1976;111 (April): 484.

11. Lieberman S: DeGraff Memorial Hospital, New York, statistics. *Same-Day Surgery* 1979;132 (January): 1.

12. Abramson D: Delaying mastectomy after outpatient breast biopsy. *American Journal of Surgery* 1976;132: 596.

13. Refined list of suggested procedures—A working draft: Ambulatory surgery project 80–003. *Michigan Hospital Association Monday Report* 1981;12 (August 10): 30.

14. *Summary Report of Graduate Medical Education National Advisory Committee to the Secretary of the Department of Health and Human Services.* US Depart of Health and Human Services, Sept 30, 1980.

15. Report on surgical services, health care financing administration. *Same-Day Surgery* 1981;5 (May 1981): 64.

Chapter 5

A Quality Assurance Program for Ambulatory Surgical Services

Sharon M. Buske, R.N., B.S.N.

THE PURPOSE OF A QUALITY ASSURANCE PROGRAM

What Is Quality Assurance?

In order to understand the concept of quality assurance as it relates to the health care setting, it is first necessary to understand the meaning of quality and quality control. *Quality* can be defined as the very best that can be consistently achieved in any situation in which the best of the extremes have been blended so as to allow for navigation of the "golden mean."

Quality control attempts to measure quality according to predetermined standards. In the manufacturing industries, quality control has long been a fundamental element. Whether the end product is perfume, plastic beverage bottles, drug preparations, or packaged food, samples are rigorously compared with minimum acceptable standards to control quality. In the health care setting, quality control is constantly practiced in the measurement and calibration of equipment and supplies. Sterilizing procedures and autoclaves, for example, are monitored frequently for efficiency; and blood gas machinery is calibrated on a predetermined schedule, as is the automated laboratory equipment. In fact, very little in the way of machinery, equipment, therapeutics, procedures, or techniques escapes the scrutiny of quality control.

Quality assurance, on the other hand, is not entirely concerned with calibration or measurement as is quality control. Instead, quality assurance deals with the reality of quality on a more cognitive level. Using as a basis the meaning of quality together with the data base collected through quality control, quality assurance strives to interpret the appropriateness of action. The practice of premedicating surgical patients with narcotics, for example, has long been considered the protocol of choice in anesthesia man-

agement; however, postoperative nausea and vomiting is often a consequence of this management. When the case is handled on an inpatient
basis, the nausea and vomiting can be managed very effectively; but
managed on an outpatient basis, the same nausea and vomiting can eventually prevent the patient's discharge and consequently lead to an overnight stay in the hospital. Obviously, what is appropriate in one set of
circumstances becomes a very significant problem in another. The questions of appropriateness of protocol, rightness of decision making, and
compatability of health care and its delivery mechanisms in a given environment comprise the territory governed by quality assurance.

Why Is Quality Assurance Needed in Health Care?

Quality control applied to a manufactured product or medical machinery
appears concrete and logical, yet quality assurance applied to a patient's
health seems abstract and confused. Quality assurance in a health care
setting, however, is as simple, concrete, and logical as quality control in
the manufacturing setting. The tendency to identify the patient as the
product of quality assurance efforts is incorrect; the quality of a patient
cannot be assured. What can be assured is the quality and appropriateness
of health care that directly or indirectly affects the state of the patient's
physical, mental, and social well-being.[1]

There is a real challenge in trying to assign values and assessment tools
to quality health care along with the concomitant accountability. Certain
resentments seem to surface. "After all," the detractors say, "dedicated
health care professionals have been giving quality care since the beginning
of medicine. And just who defines quality care? Now the Joint Commission
on Accreditation of Hospitals (JCAH) is in the picture with a new quality
assurance standard—what next?"

Although dedicated health care professionals have provided and always
will provide quality care, two facts remain. First, the interpretation of and
compliance with health care standards differs among practitioners. Although
standards for such care are established, the degree of individual interpretation and compliance varies from excellent to poor. Second, not all health
care professionals are dedicated; therefore the product, or the quality of
practice delivered, must be evaluated in terms of compliance with the
standard of care. The cycle is complete only when the unacceptable behavior is identified, assessed, changed, monitored, and documented.[1]

Who Defines Quality Care?

In defining quality care, Norma Lang implies that, besides the professions and science, society in general and the patient in particular wield a

powerful influence. Lang states, moreover, that "societal values define which end results are desirable and which are not. They also define what kinds of professional behavior and interactions are preferred over others."[2] The technical competence of health care may be impeccable, but its worth is paled by sloppy, abrupt, or insensitive delivery.

JCAH's New Standard

It is not surprising that the evaluation efforts of the JCAH have evolved into a standard that emphasizes definition of purpose, organization of effort, and correction of patient-related problems identified by objective assessment. Although hospitals have been complying with audit and evaluation requirements, the effects on improved patient care or clinical practice for the most part have not been demonstrated. Central to this issue is the fact that there is no mechanism to coordinate or integrate the findings of evaluative efforts throughout the institution.[3] As a result, during a department audit, a problem that is uncovered concerning another department goes unnoticed and unattended. Consequently, there is no improvement in patient care, despite the efforts and costs involved in problem identification.

The new JCAH standard emphasizes that the identified problems must be relative to the improvement of patient care. Moreover, these efforts must be coordinated and integrated into the institution's organization chart, which should show open lines of communication as well as where "the buck stops." The JCAH encourages creativity, innovation, and identification of problems, in addition to suggesting many identifying sources, such as financial data, utilization review findings, patient surveys or comments, and findings of hospital committees. For this reason the audit is no longer considered the only method of data collection. Exhibit 5–1 illustrates a retrospective patient care evaluation form used to document the postoperative telephone interview with the patient. Note that the form is concise and is easy for the interviewer to read and mark at a glance. If the first attempt to contact the patient is unsuccessful, a second call is made. Only two attempts are made to contact the postoperative patient. Provisions are made at the bottom of the form to reflect the calling status. Patients are not disturbed at their place of employment; instead they are called late in the afternoon or on a Saturday.

Exhibit 5–2 is an explanation of positive responses and appears on the reverse side of Exhibit 5–1. Each "yes" response requires a specific and detailed explanation with an appropriate follow up. Once completed, the retrospective patient care evaluation form becomes a part of the chart and, thus, the formal medical record.

Exhibit 5-1 Retrospective Patient Care Evaluation

SAINT FRANCIS HOSPITAL, INC.
OUTPATIENT SERVICE DEPARTMENT

RETROSPECTIVE PATIENT CARE EVALUATION: Pt. Name: _____

1. Did patient have respiratory symptoms such as congestion, wheezing, sore throat or difficulty breathing?

    ___ General   NO   YES
    ___ Other _____   (See Reverse)

2. Did patient complain of any bleeding?

                         NO   YES
                                               (See Reverse)

3. Did patient experience impairment to circulation and/or nerves such as change in color, increased pain, numbness, swelling, tingling or coldness?

    NA   NO   YES
                                               (See Reverse)

4. Did patient experience unusual pain at home?

                         NO   YES
                                               (See Reverse)

5. Did patient experience nausea and/or vomiting after discharge?

    ___ General   NO   YES
    ___ Local with sed.   (See Reverse)
    ___ Local
    ___ Block

6. Were antibiotics prescribed to be taken before surgery?

                         NO   YES
                                               (See Reverse)

7. Were antibiotics prescibed to be taken after surgery?

                         NO   YES
                                               (See Reverse)

8. Were there any signs of infection after surgery such as pus-filled or foul odor to drainage, pain, redness, swelling or fever?

                         NO   YES
                                               (See Reverse)

1st Call—Date: _____ Completed ___   2nd. Call—Date: _____ Completed ___

                   Not Completed ___   Not Completed ___

Nurse's Signature: _____ 1st Call

Nurse's Signature: _____ 2nd Call

Source: Saint Francis Hospital, Memphis, Tennessee.

Exhibit 5-2 Explanation of Positive Responses

EXPLANATION OF POSITIVE RESPONSES

1. Patient complained of respiratory symptoms including:
   ___ Congestion   ___ Sore throat   ___ Physician called
   ___ Wheezing   ___ Breathing difficulty   ___ Physician seen

   Comments: _____
   _____
   Disposition _____

2. Patient complained of postoperative bleeding:
   How long did bleeding last?_____   ___ Physician called
   How much bleeding? _____   ___ Physician seen

   Comments:_____
   _____
   Disposition:_____

3. Patient complained of impairment to circulation and/or nerves:
   ___ Change in color   ___ Increased pain   ___ Physician called
   ___ Tingling   ___ Coldness   ___ Physician seen
                     Numbness

   Comments:_____
   _____
   Disposition:_____

4. Patient complained of postoperative pain:
   ___ Mild ___ Moderate ___ Severe ___ No pain med ordered ___ Physician called
                                               ___ Physician seen
   ___ Pain med gave tolerable relief   How long did pain last before relief?_____
   ___ Pain med did not give tolerable relief   ___ Physician ordered pain med after contacting him

   Comments:_____
   _____
   Disposition:_____

5. Patient complained of nausea and/or vomiting after discharge:
   How long did nausea and/or vomiting last?_____   ___ Physician called
   ___ Further treatment required   ___ Physician seen

   Comments:_____
   _____
   Disposition:_____

6. Antibiotics were prescribed preoperatively:
   Name of med and dosage _____
   How long before surgery were these drugs taken? _____

Exhibit 5-2 continued

Comments:_____
_____

7. Antibiotics were prescribed postoperatively:
   ____ Med was taken as prescribed.
   ____ Side effects noted

   Comments:_____
   _____

8. Patient described signs and symptoms of infection:
   ___Operative site   ___Foul drainage and/   ___Redness   ___Physician
   ___Other than   or pus   ___Swelling   called
     operative site   ___Pain   ___Fever   ___Physician seen
   How long after surgery did symptoms appear?_____
                                        Med. rx'd as a result_____
   Comments:_____
   _____

   Disposition:_____

Source: Saint Francis Hospital, Memphis, Tennessee

The telephone interview is conducted between the second and fifth postoperative day and provides a wealth of valid information that can be used to assess the quality and appropriateness of care delivered. Another method of retrospective interview includes asking the patient to assume the responsibility for contacting the facility. This contact can be made by telephone or by a self-addressed, postage-paid returnable questionnaire. Whichever method is used, it is incumbent on the institution to show documentation of the effort in relation to the actual impact on patient care.[1(pp 5–6)]

COMPONENT PARTS OF A QUALITY ASSURANCE PROGRAM

The function of a quality assurance program in any health care setting is to affect patient care constructively. How the program is constructed can be as innovative and creative as necessary in order to improve patient care. There must be continuity between the efforts of the health care provider, the manufacturer, and for that matter, anyone who must assure quality. These are the component parts of any quality assurance program. The JCAH recommends that the essential components of a strong program include identifying the problem, objectively assessing the problem, implementing a solution, monitoring the effectiveness of the solution, and documenting the effectiveness of the solution.[1] In the following sections, each of these components is discussed, using the successful quality assurance program at Saint Francis Hospital in Memphis, Tennessee.

Identifying the Problem

In the ambulatory care quality assurance program at Saint Francis Hospital, a standard specified that the patient, or a responsible adult, must be aware of how to provide safe care after discharge. This standard, as well as fifteen others (see Exhibit 5–6), was incorporated into the Exhibit 5–3 questionnaire that fifty postoperative ambulatory surgical patients completed before discharge. The data was compiled, and the results indicated that one patient did not have a clear understanding of home care; thus, a problem was identified. The standard of care and the actual care did not meet the requirement of 100 percent compliance with the criteria specified. Two other problems were also identified in this fish-net approach; however, the patient's proper understanding of postoperative home care clearly took priority. This requirement complies with that of the JCAH, which calls for the priority-setting mechanism rather than a problem list. Problems need be documented only *after* they have been identified and addressed.[4]

Since an adequate understanding of home care is essential to the safety of a surgical patient who is to be discharged the same day, the scope of the problem as well as its causes had to be assessed. In this case, the problem was concurrently identified and could have been assessed in one step. One in fifty patients, however, leaves enough doubt to wonder if this patient was an exception or an indication of a future pattern of mediocre care. The question of understanding home care was incorporated into the postoperative telephone call of the next 100 patients. This approach was retrospective to data collection. The results indicated that twelve patients did not have a safe understanding of home care.

Objectively Assessing the Problem

Having fully identified the problem, the next step was to assess its causes. A meeting was held with the staff, and the problem presented. Each staff member was interviewed as to the content of discharge instructions, amount of time spent with the patient, and problems associated with giving discharge instructions. The results indicated that the content was subject to a great deal of interpretation. The amount of time spent with each patient averaged less than five minutes, and the problems associated

Exhibit 5-3 Concurrent Review

TO THE SURGERY PATIENT: Please take a minute to answer the following questions. We are trying to evaluate just how effectively we take care of you.

		YES	NO
1.	Were you taken care of promptly on arrival?	___	___
2.	Were the forms that you were asked to sign explained to you?	___	___
3.	Were the procedures that the nurse performed explained to you?	___	___
4.	Did you feel as if you were being cared for efficiently and competently?	___	___
5.	Did you feel free to ask questions?	___	___
6.	Were your questions answered to your satisfaction?	___	___
7.	Were signs and symptoms of possible problems that may occur at home explained to you?	___	___
8.	Do you understand how to take care of yourself at home?	___	___
9.	If problems occur at home, do you know who to call?	___	___
10.	If you had take-home prescriptions, were they explained to you?	___	___
11.	Was your privacy provided for and respected?	___	___
12.	Were your valuables, clothes and other belongings returned to you in good condition?	___	___
13.	Was financial responsibility for your operation made clear to you by the receptionist?	___	___
14.	Did you see any practice which you felt would put your safety in jeopardy? If "Yes," comment below.	___	___
15.	Did you feel that you were treated with respect and courtesy at all times?	___	___

Other Comments:

                              Thanks:
                              Outpatient Services

Source: Sharon M. Buske, "Quality Assurance in the Ambulatory Care Setting," *Tennessee Hospital Times* 22, No. 5 (June 1981): 4.

---

with giving the instructions ranged from not having enough staff to leaving before they could be given the instructions.

Implementing a Solution

Implementing a solution began with a second meeting of the nursing staff and the chief anesthesiologist. The staff decided that there should be some standardization in postoperative discharge instructions to patients.

To ensure this standardization and to guarantee that once home the patient remembered the instructions, the data was incorporated into a written form, a copy of which the patient took home. The form, shown in Exhibits 5–4 and 5–5, was developed and submitted for approval by the medical staff and administration. In-service education followed in order to teach the staff how to use and complete the form. An addition to the nursing staff was made to maximize the quality of time spent with the patient in giving discharge instructions. Several in-service programs were scheduled to point out effective teaching techniques and common pitfalls to avoid. A postpartum mother, for example, cannot understand a nurse's instruction if she cannot hear the nurse because her infant is crying in her lap. In this case, the instructions could be given to the father or other responsible relative outside the room. Should the mother be the only one present, the nurse would be well advised to wait until the child quieted down before proceeding.

Monitoring the Effectiveness of the Solution

The postoperative instruction form was implemented. The next step was to monitor its effectiveness in solving the problem. At the end of one month, patients were sampled again for appropriate understanding of home care. The result was 100 percent compliance with the stated standard. With the desired results having been achieved, the next step was to validate sustained results. After one year, fifty patients were interviewed concurrently and fifty patients were interviewed retrospectively. In both cases the results indicated 100 percent compliance with the standard.

Documenting the Effectiveness of the Solution

Appropriate documentation substantiated the effectiveness of the effort. Should the monitoring have proven that the implemented solution was ineffective, the process would have reverted to the implementation phase.

QUALITY ASSURANCE IN THE AMBULATORY SURGICAL SETTING

The Patient As Active Participant in Care

Ambulatory surgery is an aggressive arena for modern health care delivery. The patient and family are expected to follow very specific instructions both preoperatively and postoperatively. In contrast to the inpatient—

Exhibit 5-4 Postoperative Discharge Instruction Form

POSTOPERATIVE   SAINT FRANCIS HOSPITAL, INC.
INSTRUCTIONS   OUTPATIENT SERVICES
                    5959 Park Avenue ● Memphis, Tennessee

YOU ARE URGED TO FOLLOW CAREFULLY THE FOLLOWING INSTRUCTIONS:

_____Make an appointment to see your physician in/on _____.

_____Observe the operative areas for signs of excessive bleeding. (Slow general oozing that saturates the dressing completely or frank bright red bleeding.) In either case, apply pressure to the area, elevate it if possible and contact your physician at once!

_____Observe the affected extremity for circulation or nerve impairment:

    Change in color   Coldness
    Numbness or tingling   Increased pain

If any of these signs or symptoms are present, call your physician at once!

_____Observe the operative areas for signs of infection:

    Increased pain   Swelling
    Redness   Foul odor

These signs and symptoms usually become apparent in 36 to 48 hours. If present, contact your physician.

_____Keep the operative areas clean and dry. Do not remove the dressing unless instructed to do so by your physician.

_____Keep the operative site elevated for the next 12 to 24 hours.

_____Apply ice to the operative site as directed.

_____Avoid stress to the suture line such as pulling, pushing, etc.

_____May change the nasal tip dressing as needed and as demonstrated.

_____Avoid sneezing or blowing the nose.

_____Keep water out of the ears.

REGARDING ANESTHESIA:

If you had general anesthesia or local anesthesia with sedation, please pay particular attention to the following instructions:

1. Do not drink alcoholic beverages including beer for 24 hours. Alcohol enhances the effects of anesthesia and sedation.

2. Do not drive a motor vehicle, operate machinery or power tools for 24 hours. If a child, no bicycle riding, skateboards, gym sets, etc., for 24 hours.

3. Do not make any important decisions or sign important papers for 24 hours.

4. You may experience lightheadedness, dizziness and sleepiness following surgery. Please DO NOT STAY ALONE. A responsible adult should be with you for this 24-hour period.

5. Rest at home with moderate activity as tolerated. It may not be necessary to go to bed; however, it is important to rest for 24 hours following general anesthesia.

6. Progress slowly to a regular diet unless your physician has instructed you otherwise. Start with liquids such as soft drinks, then soup and crackers gradually working up to solid foods.

7. Certain anesthetics and pain medications may produce nausea and vomiting in certain individuals. If nausea becomes a problem at home, call your physician. In the meantime, rest or sleep on your side to avoid accidentally inhaling material that you may vomit.

Exhibit 5-4 continued

REGARDING MEDICATIONS:

1. If your physician ordered pain medication, please take it as directed. Do not drive a motor vehicle, operate machinery or power tools while taking this medication.
2. Check with your physician regarding medications which you were taking prior to surgery.

POSTOPERATIVE TELEPHONE CALL:

A representative from the Outpatient Service Department may call you by telephone a few days after surgery. Do not be alarmed. This is a routine call to find out how you are progressing after your surgery.

If you should experience difficulty in breathing, bleeding that you feel is excessive, persistent nausea or vomiting, any pain that is unusual, swelling or fever, please call your physician. If you find that you cannot contact your physician but feel that your signs and symptoms warrant a physician's attention, go to an Emergency Room which is closest to you.

OTHER INSTRUCTIONS: _____

_____

_____

I hereby accept, understand, and can verbalize these instructions:

Witness:_____ Patient or Guardian:_____

Date:_____ Relationship to Patient:_____

Source: Saint Francis Hospital, Memphis, Tennessee.

whose water pitcher is removed by staff personnel the night before surgery—the ambulatory surgical patient plays an active role in the prescribed care. Postoperatively, the patient is sent, not to the skilled eyes and hands of nurses for twenty-four hours, but home to family members who must be given enough information to make rational judgments on behalf of the patient's safety. The physician relies heavily on the active cooperation of the patient and family in order to deliver the contracted care. The nurses in the ambulatory surgical setting should be highly sensitive to patients' attitudes and apprehensions and deft at preparing the patient and family for active, skillful home care.

One Missing Element

There is one traditional element that is missing in the modern approach to health care delivery: time. Patients who previously had spent a minimum of twenty-four hours or more in the hospital for surgery may be in and out

Exhibit 5-5 Postoperative Discharge Instruction Form

CHARGES

AMBULATORY SURGERY

The surgical Price Schedule for Ambulatory Surgery patients includes the following: surgical suite and supplies, recovery room, outpatient preparation and postoperative observation, **routine** laboratory studies, anesthesia supplies, medications, radiology done in operating room and pathology. This price **DOES NOT INCLUDE** charges for prosthetic devices, surgeon's fees, anesthesiologist or anesthetist fees which may be billed by the hospital, radiologist fees or take-home drugs. You can expect a statement of these charges in approximately 2 weeks. If you have insurance that covers your surgery, we will file a claim with your insurance company for reimbursement. If you do not have insurance or your insurance will not cover the charges, you are expected to make payment within 15 days after receipt of the mailed statement. For information concerning these charges, contact the Saint Francis Hospital Business Office, 5959 Park Avenue, P.O. Box 171808, Memphis, Tennessee 38117, telephone 901-765-1850. Direct questions regarding Medicare or Medicaid to 901-765-1877.

X-RAY CHARGES

Not included in the x-ray charges are professional fees for services by the Memphis Physician's Radiological Group. In the event that an x-ray is necessary in surgery, this group of radiologists will give a final reading. You will receive a separate bill for their professional services. For information, contact Memphis Physician's Radiological Group, 6005 Park Avenue, Suite 306, Memphis, Tennessee 38138, telephone 901-761-2160.

FOR INFORMATION CONCERNING SERVICES IN THE OUTPATIENT SERVICE DEPARTMENT, PLEASE CONTACT THE OUTPATIENT DEPARTMENT DIRECTOR AT 765-2165.

IF YOU HAVE ANY COMPLIMENTS OR COMPLAINTS, CALL THE SAINT FRANCIS HOSPITAL PATIENT REPRESENTATIVE SERVICE AT 765-1833.

Source: Saint Francis Hospital, Memphis, Tennessee.

---

in less than four hours. As a consequence, there simply is less time to observe the patient, document the care given, prepare postoperative instructions, handle financial snags, prepare for the next patient, and identify problems.

Quality Assurance Based on Patient Outcomes

How can the quality of a patient's health care be properly evaluated when the length of stay is measured in hours and minutes instead of in days and weeks? Joseph Gonella, M.D., believes that "patient outcomes should therefore be the primary focus of quality assurance programs."[5] At Saint Francis Hospital, sixteen expected patient outcomes have been developed and are consistent with the philosophy of the hospital in general and the Ambulatory Care Department in particular (see Exhibit 5–6).[6] In addition to the specific outcomes desired, standards of behavior were developed for each outcome in order to assure consistency of the quality and quantity of care delivered. The eighth expected patient outcome, for example, states: "That the patient suffered no undue anxiety because the procedure was not explained." The standard of behavior developed to ensure that this outcome is realized reads as follows:

> As well as preparing the patient physically for the procedure, the right to emotional preparation through information and instruction is also recognized. Qualified personnel are available in both the outpatient service department, as well as in other departments, to explain the steps of the procedure.
>
> The patient who goes to surgery will be told what to expect before and after the operation, where the relative will be waiting and what to expect on return to the outpatient service department. The patient will be directly asked if there are further questions.
>
> These actions are based on the premise that fear of the unknown causes anxiety, which is detrimental to the physical and psychological well-being of the patient who is to undergo a surgical experience. This fear and anxiety are preventable through effective preparation in the outpatient service department.
>
> Recognizing that the family members of the surgical patient are a means of support, we include them in the surgical experience by keeping them in touch with progress in the operating room. For example, the family is notified by outpatient service personnel when returning to the outpatient service department. They are also included in discharge teaching, which is documented on the outpatient service department's after-care sheet.
>
> Moreover, the family members will be told where to wait and advised not to leave for breakfast, etc., until they have spoken to the physician, who usually calls on the telephone. Relatives are considered an active and responsible part of the patient's overall surgical experience before, during and more importantly after discharge. They are encouraged to stay with the patient both before and after the surgical experience.[7]

Exhibit 5-6 Expected Patient Outcomes

OUTPATIENT SERVICES DEPARTMENT

I. EXPECTED PATIENT OUTCOMES:

The patient who upon a physician's order submits to a procedure directed by the Saint Francis Hospital Outpatient Services Department can expect to be discharged from the department with the following assurances:

1. That the patient understands each form that requires a signature and why the signature or that of a responsible party is necessary.
2. That the patient understands who and how financial responsibility for the procedure will be handled and who generates the bills if other than the hospital.
3. That the patient's safety home is assured when appropriate by having a responsible person available to provide transportation.
4. That the procedures were coordinated in such a way as to provide for accuracy of scheduling as well as efficiency of time.
5. That the procedure was performed safely and accurately by qualified personnel and only according to the physician's specific instructions and plan of care.
6. That qualified personnel were available at all times to answer questions.
7. That the patient's privacy has been provided for and respected.
8. That the patient suffered no undue anxiety because the procedure was not explained.
9. That precautions to insure the patient's safety in the Outpatient Services Department have been practiced at all times.
10. That should a sudden change in the patient's condition occur requiring emergency intervention, trained personnel and necessary equipment were readily available.
11. That the patient's valuables and belongings have been kept in safekeeping until discharge.
12. That the patient understand what the prescriptions are for, when to take them and precautions to observe when taking certain drugs which affect sensory-motor function.
13. That the patient and responsible party understand exactly how to take responsibility for home care.
14. That the patient and responsible party know exactly what untoward signs and symptoms to look for after discharge which would alert them to possible problems.
15. That the patient knows who to call for help if untoward signs and/or symptoms become apparent.
16. That the patient was treated as a unique individual with the respect and dignity which is recognized as a fundamental right of every patient entering Saint Francis Hospital.

Source: Sharon M. Buske, "Quality Assurance in the Ambulatory Care Setting," *Tennessee Hospital Times* 22, no. 5 (June 1981): 4; and Joan Jackson, ed., "Patient Outcomes Shape Quality Assurance Programs," *Same-Day Surgery* 5, no. 1 (January 1981): 11.

An Effective Program Should Include a Plan

In order to provide a consistently effective quality assurance program, the JCAH suggests a written plan in which the goals and standards of care are stated. The plan, moreover, should be comprehensive enough to cover all aspects of the health care delivery mechanism in any ambulatory surgical setting. It should be flexible enough to be innovative and realistic enough to be practical.[8] The JCAH, for example, requires a review of ambulatory surgical patients needing unplanned postoperative admission.[9] Exhibit 5-7 illustrates the format and results of a review done at Saint Francis Hospital on unplanned surgical admissions. The character of the results reflects its ongoing nature.

Cooperative Effort Stressed

Problem solving, central to the concept of quality assurance, is a cooperative effort involving clear, open lines of communication. *Hospital Peer Review*, for example, documents a case involving two surgical patients whose identities were confused by hospital personnel. The error was noted only after both surgical procedures had begun. In addition to assigning blame specifically to two anesthesiologists—and generally to seventeen other staff members working in two operating rooms—public health officials indicated a "total breakdown in the system of checks and balances set up to ensure proper patient identifications."[10]

The quality assurance plan should outline the relationship of ambulatory surgery review efforts to other departments within the institution. The plan, moreover, should indicate the mechanism by which quality assurance activities affect the vertical responsibility within the medical staff, administration, and governing board. Figure 5-1 is a sample of one of many approaches to designating mechanisms of communication and accountability. The entire plan should be reassessed annually in light of its effectiveness, appropriateness and currency. Moreover, the impact on patient care must be documented in order to validate any effective quality assurance program.[1] (pp 5-6)

The Quality of Caring

In the final analysis, it is the quality of caring that is essential. Although acknowledged standards of care and practice can be measured, we cannot guarantee excellence of caring from these standards alone; the latter must come from within each individual. A truly effective quality assurance program will guarantee not only appropriateness of care and technical excellence but also that "every patient, regardless of the extent of his physical or psychological disability, has a right to be treated with a respect consonant with his dignity as a person."[11]

Figure 5-1 Organizational Chart

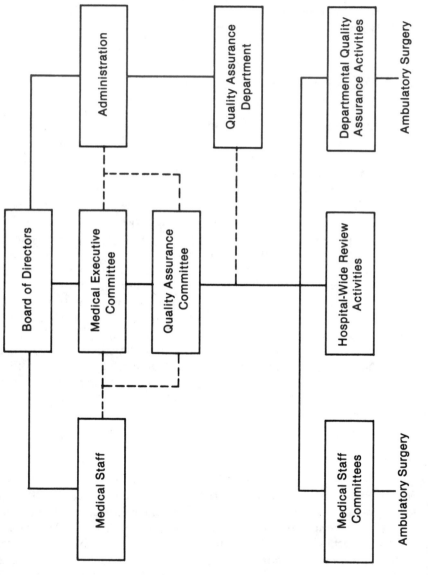

Source: Saint Francis Hospital, Memphis, Tennessee.

Exhibit 5-7 Example of Review Format

REVIEW OF UNPLANNED ADMISSION TO THE HOSPITAL FOLLOWING
SURGERY DONE ON AN AMBULATORY BASIS

I. Concern of Study:

   A. To identify the extent and causes necessitating unplanned admission to the hospital following ambulatory surgery done through the Outpatient Services Department of Saint Francis Hospital.

II. Results of Study:

   A. Extent of Unplanned Admission
      1. Of the 1,950 surgical cases done through the Outpatient Services Department from 1/1/80 through 12/31/80, 13 patients were admitted for further observation.
      2. This represents a .6 percent admission rate for unforeseen complications.

   B. Causes of Unplanned Admission
      1. Three patients were admitted for nausea and vomiting, one of which was also very sleepy.
      2. Two patients were admitted for unstable vital signs, particularly hypotension.
      3. Two patients were admitted due to severe pain.
      4. One patient requested admission.
      5. One patient developed a hematoma which necessitated a return to surgery and evacuation of same.
      6. One patient's physician requested 24-hour observation for bleeding after the removal of a rectal polyp.
      7. One patient was too sleepy to discharge.
      8. One patient required additional and more extensive surgery.
      9. One patient developed hoarseness, coughing and chest pain.

III. Problems Identified:

   A. Seven of the 13 cases admitted appear to be the result of anesthesia related problems with nausea and vomiting being the most consistently repeated offenders. (12 of the 13 patients reviewed were done under general anesthesia.)

   B. The remaining five situations requiring eventual admission appear to have no common thread of correlation other than that they could not have been anticipated preoperatively.
      1. Action Recommended:
      Complete a study of 100 adult and 100 pediatric ambulatory surgical patients done under general anesthesia:

      Document and compare the following:
         1. age
         2. weight
         3. procedure
         4. anesthesiologist
         5. anesthesia risk
         6. preoperative medications

Exhibit 5-7 continued

> 7. anesthetics used
> 8. duration of anesthesia
> 9. length of recovery room stay
> 10. medications used during recovery
> 11. length of outpatient observation stay
> 12. medications used during outpatient observations
> 13. incidence of anesthesia related problems during outpatient observation
> 14. incidence of anesthesia related problems after discharge
>
> The purpose of this study will be to collect a data base in order to profile and identify the present anesthesia management of the ambulatory surgical patient. This study will be done in cooperation with the Anesthesia Medical Staff Committee to whom the data will be submitted for review and recommendations. The data will concurrently be submitted to the required committees in the usual fashion.
>
> IV. Action Taken:
>
> A. A study of 100 adult and 100 pediatric ambulatory surgical patients undergoing general anesthesia will be completed by Sharon M. Buske, R.N. with the results submitted to the Anesthesia Medical Staff Committee for review and recommendations.
>
> V. Followup Evaluation:
>
> A. Study of 100 adult and 100 pediatric patients' charts to be completed by September, 1981.
>
> *Source:* Saint Francis Hospital, Memphis, Tennessee.

REFERENCES

1. Redman RR (ed): New JCAH quality assurance standard for hospitals. *Perspective on Accreditation,* May–June 1979, p 5.

2. Davidson S, et al: *PSRO Utilization and Audit in Patient Care.* St Louis, CV Mosby, 1976, pp 20–22.

3. Redman, RR (ed): New QA standard approved. *Perspectives on Accreditation,* May–June, 1979, p 2.

4. Redman RR (ed): Documentation requirements for QA. *Perspectives on Accreditation,* September–October 1980, p 6.

5. Gonella J, MD: Toward an effective system of ambulatory health care evaluation. *Quarterly Review Bulletin* 1977;3 (October): 8.

6. Jackson (ed.): Special report: Same-day surgery—1980. *Same-Day Surgery* 1981;5 (January): 11.

7. Buske SM, RN: Quality assurance. *Same-Day Surgery* 1980;4 (February–March): 18.

8. Redman RR (ed): An explanation of the new quality assurance standard. *Perspectives on Accreditation,* May–June 1979, pp 7–9.

9. Joint Commission on Accreditation of Hospitals: *Accreditation Manual for Hospitals, 1980 Edition.* Chicago, Joint Commission on Accreditation of Hospitals, 1979, p 69.

10. Benson, DB (ed): QA: A factor in switched surgeries. *Hospital Peer Review* 1980;5 (November 1980): 129.

11. United States Catholic Conference: *Ethical and religious directives for Catholic health facilities.* Washington, DC, United States Catholic Conference, 1977, p 3.

Chapter 6

Hospital-Based Ambulatory Surgery: Two Case Studies

James O. Jonassen, AIA

One of the first decisions in planning and designing an ambulatory surgical facility is the selection of the basic model type to be followed. Generically, the models can be divided into five types: (1) a freestanding, independent unit not physically connected to or affiliated with a hospital; (2) a freestanding unit associated with but not physically connected to a hospital; (3) a freestanding facility associated with and physically connected to a hospital; (4) a facility owned and physically integrated into a hospital but not part of the hospital's inpatient surgical suite; (5) a facility owned and physically integrated with a hospital and its inpatient surgical suite.

The selection of one of these models is dependent on the objectives of the sponsor and the services that will be delivered in the suite. On one hand, a totally freestanding, independent unit may be able to deliver some surgical procedures at lower cost because of a lower overhead burden. On the other hand, a hospital-integrated unit that is part of the major inpatient suite may be able to take care of even more complex cases on an outpatient basis because of the ready availability of backup staff and equipment that might become necessary if the case proves to be more difficult than anticipated.

The facilities discussed in this chapter represent two different models of hospital-associated ambulatory surgical suites. One of these is inte-

I wish to thank Ms. Barbara Levinski, R.N., Clinical Supervisor for Surgery at the Swedish Hospital Medical Center, Mr. Donn Berg, Director of Surgery, and Ms. Nancy Duncan, Director of Admitting at Virginia Mason Medical Center, for their generous assistance in evaluation of these suites as well as for their work during the planning. I would further like to thank Dr. Allan Lobb, Executive Director at the Swedish Hospital Medical Center, and Mr. Donald Olson, Administrator of Virginia Mason Hospital, for their permission to review the suites with their staff; and finally I would like to thank Ms. Keri Dean, my Administrative Assistant, for her help in organizing this paper.

grated with a hospital and is a part of the hospital's inpatient surgical suite. The other model is associated with a hospital but is physically freestanding except for a connecting bridge.

BASIC GOALS OF AMBULATORY SURGERY

Patient convenience is one of the important goals of developing an ambulatory surgical facility. Convenience is achieved by reducing the length of time patients need to be away from their families and jobs, and, in some cases, by providing greater flexibility in scheduling surgery on an ambulatory rather than inpatient basis.

Convenience to physicians is also an important consideration. Physician convenience can be achieved in ambulatory surgery when physicians can schedule a major block of short surgical cases in a concentrated time and when the flow of patients through the suite is easy to control.

Reduced cost to the patient is another major goal of developing ambulatory surgical suites. This goal is often the primary focus in discussing ambulatory surgery. Cost reductions can be achieved in several ways. The primary reduction in cost, and the one that most affects the patient, is the elimination of a hospital stay (not including the patient's time in the operating room). Eliminating one or two days of hospitalization can amount to a savings of two to six hundred dollars (in 1981), and that savings alone can cut the bills of some surgical patients in half. In some cases, additional cost savings can be realized through lower charges for operating or recovery room time, or by reducing the time required in the operating room. Generally, these latter savings are less significant and are highly dependent on the basic model type and the resulting overhead cost of the facility. A third means of reducing cost may be brought about through reduction of the required amount of preoperative laboratory testing.

CRITERIA FOR SELECTION OF MODEL TYPE

Other major criteria in selecting a basic model and design for an ambulatory surgical facility frequently relate to the specific needs of the sponsor. Some hospital sponsors, for example, may choose a freestanding ambulatory surgical unit because it provides a means of increasing total surgical capacity when there is no reasonable opportunity to expand an inpatient suite in a contiguous way. Others may choose a surgical facility that integrates outpatient and inpatient surgery because it is the only model that accommodates physical constraints.

CRITERIA FOR DESIGN

Regardless of the basic model chosen, major criteria for the internal design of the ambulatory surgical unit generally involve patient access and flow, operating room support, special requirements for pediatrics, physician access, and peak case loading.

Patient Access and Flow

A basic goal of an ambulatory surgical facility is to provide patients with more convenience and lower costs than is possible when surgery is performed on an inpatient basis. The way in which patient-facility interaction is handled is one of the paramount design considerations affecting this goal. The flow of patients through the facility can be broken down into seven stages: prearrival, arrival, preparation, induction, recovery, postrecovery, and discharge.

The prearrival procedure influences the unit design particularly in the reception area. Patients are often instructed to come to the ambulatory surgical facility on the day preceding surgery to receive dietary and arrival instructions, and to verify that preadmission laboratory tests have been completed satisfactorily. This instruction mandates that the reception area be staffed for extended hours to accommodate working patients. Depending on the extent of preadmission testing or examination, an examining or consultation room adjacent to the reception area may be needed.

Patients are usually requested to arrive at the ambulatory surgery reception desk on the day of surgery 1 to 1½ hours before the scheduled surgery. This requirement allows for further verification that preadmission testing has been completed, and, more important, for ample time to make last minute schedule adjustments to assure rapid and continuous patient flow.

When a patient arrives, a check is made to ensure that an escort will be present during discharge. These two requirements—extended waiting time and presence of an escort—influence waiting space requirements and create a significant waiting area peak load in the earlier schedule hours.

Shortly before surgery, the patient is transferred to a preoperative preparation area. The patient proceeds to a dressing area to undress and don a surgical gown. This procedure necessitates a lockable dressing cubicle where the patient's clothes can remain during the procedure, or provision of a clothing locker separate from the dressing cubicle. The key to the locker or dressing cubicle is usually attached to the patient's chart. The preoperative preparation is sometimes performed in two different areas. The first is a curtained waiting area (separating male and female patients). When this area is provided, it becomes the major staging area for controlling the facility's schedule. The second area is the preparation area itself. Here medications are administered, and shaving and cleansing are performed. A last minute blood test (hematocrit) or urinalysis is also performed here. In some cases, an intravenous fluid may be started as well. In such a case, the patient must be placed on a stretcher or a portable surgical table top.

Usually the patient is walked from the preparation area to the operating room and then climbs onto the operating table. Anesthetic induction almost always takes place in the operating room.

Following the surgical procedure, the patient is transferred to a recovery area and remains there until either totally prepared to go home or until stabilized and conscious. In many cases, the stabilized, conscious patient is transferred to a postrecovery observation area and stays there until well enough for discharge and until the escort has arrived. Some facilities provide still another area for patient postrecovery—a dressed waiting area (the patient is dressed in street clothes and ready for discharge).

Variations in the sequence of patient events are the major program variants that affect the physical development of ambulatory surgery suite designs.

Operating Room Support

It is sometimes thought that the procedure for distributing materials in and cleaning the operating room in an ambulatory surgical unit can be significantly simpler than those for an inpatient surgical suite because of the less complex case mix and higher turnover. The opposite may be true, however. Due to the necessity for high turnover and reasonable asepsis control, it is extremely important that the supply system be very responsive in supplying the operating room, and that the system for cleaning the room between cases be both fast and effective.

In a community hospital inpatient surgical suite, the average length of procedure may vary from one hour to over two hours, depending on the complexity of cases handled. This variance means that there are only two to four turnovers per operating room per day. Ten to fifteen minutes more or less in turnover time therefore has relatively little influence on the overall utilization of the operating room. In the case of an ambulatory surgical procedure, however, the average length of procedure may vary from thirty to fifty minutes, allowing seven to ten turnovers per operating room per day. Obviously, in this case a small difference in turnaround time can have a significant influence on overall operating room utilization.

Special Requirements for Pediatrics

If an ambulatory surgical suite is to serve a significant number of pediatric patients, special requirements for pediatrics become critical to the design of the suite. One factor is the extent to which the parent will accompany the child through the process. Another important consideration is the degree of separation between adults and children in waiting, holding, and recovery areas. In the ideal case of unlimited resources, it is desirable to separate completely pediatric and adult patients at every step in the process. There are three reasons why children and adults should be separated in this setting. First, children should be placed in a playful, friendly, child-oriented environment, and should not be exposed to a roomful of adult strangers in this stressful situation. Second, parents should be allowed to accompany their children through as much of the process as possible in order to provide reassurance and to assist the staff in reducing the children's fright. In a mixed area, this practice would invade the privacy of the adult patients. Third, adults should not be subjected to the unsettling noise of children during a time of significant stress and concern.

Physician Access

To be effective for physicians, an ambulatory surgical suite should allow adequate block scheduling time so that a series of short-duration cases can be scheduled at contiguous times. The design should also enable physicians to enter and leave the site rapidly so as to avoid or facilitate encounters with the patient's family as required. Easy access to recovery and postrecovery holding areas should also be provided to allow physicians to check on the condition of their patients with minimum effort.

Peak Case Loading

In inpatient surgical suites, peak case loading typically takes place at the early part of the week, allowing for recovery within the week and discharge by the weekend. Ambulatory surgical facilities also have peak case loading patterns. Peak loading for ambulatory surgery, however, tends to be late in the week (Thursday and Friday). The patients themselves like to schedule surgery so as to have the weekend at home for recovery and to minimize loss of working time.

CASE STUDIES

The following sections describe two ambulatory surgical suites designed at approximately the same time for hospitals in the same western city in the United States. They represent different model types. The first type (Case Study A) is a freestanding, hospital-affiliated unit connected to the hospital by a pedestrian bridge that crosses a street. The second type (Case Study B) is a unit that is also hospital affiliated but that is integrated into the hospital and the hospital's inpatient surgical suite.

James O. Jonassen was the architect for both these ambulatory surgical facilities. In each case the surgical suite supervisor and key staff surgeons participated extensively in the programming, planning, and design of these units.

Case Study A

The facility in Case Study A is owned by and located on the campus of a major medical center. The hospital of the medical center has approximately six hundred beds. Planning for the ambulatory surgery facility began in 1972 and was subject to the then-current certificate-of-need law because it was developed through the expenditure of hospital funds.

The model type chosen for this facility was a freestanding location connected to the hospital by a bridge. There were several reasons for selecting this model. First, the hospital was experiencing extremely high utilization of its major inpatient suite, and alternatives for expansion of that suite would have been difficult to accomplish and more costly to implement than the development of a freestanding ambulatory facility. Second, the hospital was in the process of developing a new, second medical office building on the campus. This building would be linked to the hospital and would therefore provide an excellent location for an ambulatory surgical facility. Third, this was the first major implementation of ambulatory surgery at the medical center, and the belief was that physicians would be more likely to accept the facility if it was freestanding.

The medical building location also would provide direct access for the sixty-five hospital staff physicians who would be tenants of the building. All-weather access also would be available for another hundred staff physicians through the bridge connection to the hospital and through the hospital's connection to its first medical office building. The new medical office building would have its front door on one of the busier, commercially oriented streets in the neighborhood. It would have high visibility and relatively easy access for patients. Patient parking would be provided on a surface lot across the street from the building and in hospital-owned parking garages two and four city blocks away. The facility opened in the fall of 1975.

Capacity and Size

In terms of capacity and size, this ambulatory surgical facility has two segments: a normal ambulatory surgery of five operating rooms, and an endoscopy suite that includes four treatment-examination rooms. The ambulatory surgery portion of this suite has a total of 12,670 gross square feet. The endoscopy suite has 980 gross square feet.

An analysis of existing inpatient workload during preparation of the certificate-of-need application indicated that approximately 290 of the annual inpatient surgery cases at the hospital at that time were candidates for ambulatory surgery. It was anticipated that at least half would actually be performed on an ambulatory basis if a facility were available. The anticipated initial case load of the suite was seven cases per day, and it was forecast that the load would double within the first two years of operation.

Suite Arrangement

As indicated in Figure 6-1, the patient arrives at the suite, which is on an upper floor of the medical office building, by means of the building elevators. Signs direct the patient to the reception and waiting areas of the ambulatory surgical suite (see Exhibit 6-1). Adjacent to this waiting area are a consultation room, simple laboratory and blood drawing area, and the endoscopy suite.

From the waiting area, the patient proceeds to a passage near the elevators that leads to the dressing and locker areas. Next is a preoperative holding area where final preparation takes place (blood pressure, patient weight, history, temperature, procedure description). There is no holding or staging of patients here. From the preoperative area, a nurse walks the patient to one of the five operating rooms, where the patient climbs onto an operating table.

Following surgery, the patient is wheeled from the operating room to the recovery area. This area includes a room for isolation and a separate area for pediatric patient recovery. The patient is held in the recovery area until completely recovered and ready for discharge.

During the recovery process, the patient is transferred from a stretcher to an upright chair when fully conscious and feeling well enough to sit. This transfer takes place in the same space. When the patient is fully recovered, family or an escort are allowed to join the patient. The patient is given discharge instructions in this space and sent back to the dressing room. From there, the patient goes home. If a general anesthetic has been

Figure 6-1 Floor Plan for Case Study A Ambulatory Surgical Facility

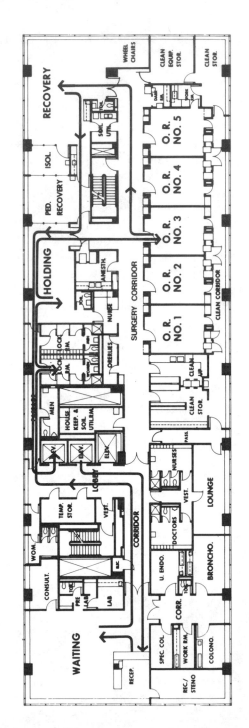

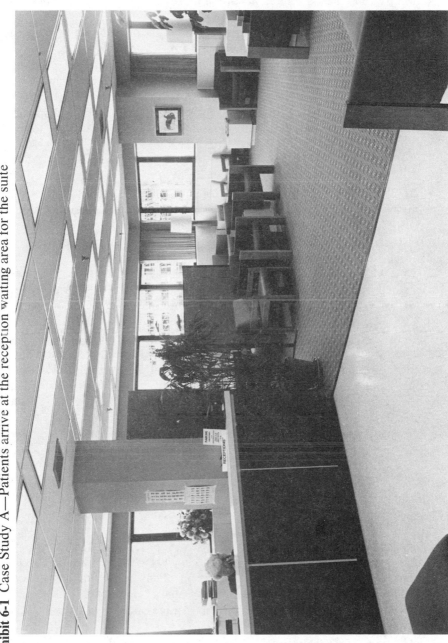

Exhibit 6-1 Case Study A—Patients arrive at the reception waiting area for the suite

administered, the patient is accompanied to the building entrance by a nurse.

Staff dressing, locker, and lounge facilities are provided at the entrance to the suite. Materials are supplied to the operating rooms through pass-through cabinets located off a clean dedicated supply corridor (see Exhibit 6-2). Equipment for each case is assembled and set into the cabinet by the operating suite supply staff. Soiled materials are removed from the rooms on the surgery corridor and taken to the soiled utility room for disposal or to the clean-up room for reprocessing.

Postoccupancy Evaluation

This ambulatory surgical facility has been evaluated several times since its initial occupancy, most recently after it had been in operation for six years. Significant findings of these evaluations include some unexpected constraints on balanced utilization and changes in methods of operation from those anticipated during the design process.

The preoperative patient flow is working as intended, and the areas designed for it have proven adequate for the most part. The waiting area, however, which accommodates thirty-five people, is pressed for space on peak load days, primarily due to the coincidence of peak load in endoscopy and surgery. An exception is the preoperative preparation (holding) area. Experience in this area suggests that it would be desirable to provide two smaller, more private areas for patient preparation. Since patients are not being held here for any length of time, the large space is not needed; but because the information exchange between patient, anesthesiologist, and nurse is very sensitive, more privacy would be appropriate.

The operating rooms are smaller than rooms in the hospital's inpatient surgical suite (240 net square feet versus 400 net square feet). This size was studied in detail during the design process and to date has proven to work very well. The operating rooms have also accommodated some portable equipment not originally anticipated, such as lasers (see Exhibit 6-3). Some procedures, however, currently being considered as candidates for the ambulatory suite may require additional portable equipment—such as microscopes for eye procedures, arthroscopes, and C-arm x-ray equipment— which will make these rooms very crowded. The need for additional portable equipment as time goes on seems as inevitable a development in ambulatory surgery as it is in inpatient surgery. This situation creates the need for more equipment storage space as well as a larger operating room.

The recovery area has proven to be utilized much differently than anticipated. This result is largely due to the growth of programs making use of

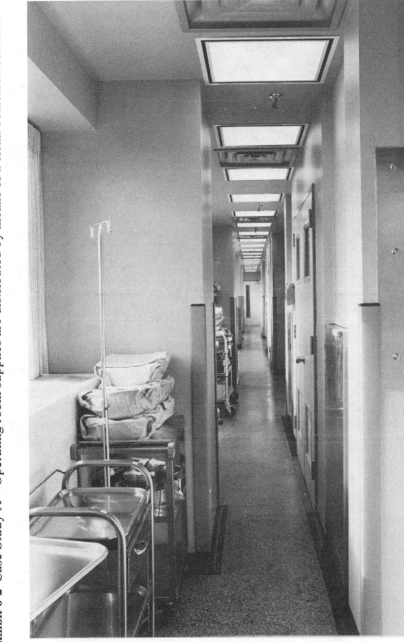

Exhibit 6-2 Case Study A—Operating room supplies are distributed by means of a clean dedicated corridor.

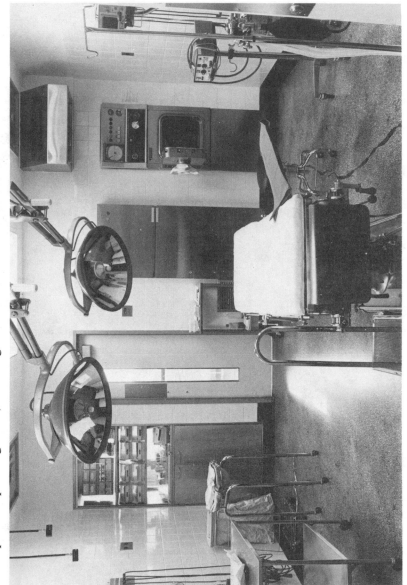

Exhibit 6-3 Case Study A—The operating rooms have most of the equipment normally found in a general inpatient operating room, including the flash autoclave in the corner.

the suite, which was not anticipated at the time of design. Liver biopsy patients from the endoscopy suite are held in the recovery area for long periods of time. Pain clinic patients receive blocks here, including time-consuming differential spinal blocks, which can take several hours. The recovery area can accommodate fourteen patients, which is believed to be adequate for the five operating rooms; however, it is not adequate to accommodate the non-surgical workload as well.

The flow of patients through the recovery area has also been redefined since the suite opened. A three-stage process is now used. In stage one, the patient, having recently been wheeled in from the operating room, is still asleep. This stage lasts an average of one-half hour.

After awakening, the patient is moved to another part of the room (stage two). The nursing staff keeps patients at this location until they are able to sit up, take some liquids, and go to the bathroom. This stage lasts forty-five to sixty minutes. From here, the patient is moved off the stretcher and into a chair, remaining there until fully alert and ready for discharge (see Exhibit 6-4). Family is allowed to join the patient during this period (stage three), which usually lasts twenty minutes to one-half hour. To accommodate this flow, the separate pediatric recovery area—which was deemed dispensable since the anticipated pediatric case load did not develop—has been removed to form one large area through which the patient moves sequentially from right to left.

The surgical workload in the suite approximated the forecast for the first two years of operation, and by 1981 the average number of cases per day had reached twenty-three. Based on the average case length (approximately forty minutes) and an average turnaround time (approximately twenty minutes), the suite was operating at slightly over 61 percent utilization, based on a 7½ hour day. There were significant peak loads, however, on Thursdays and Fridays, when the caseload averaged thirty to thirty-five cases, or approximately 87 percent utilization. The recovery-area constraints mentioned earlier were limiting increases in capacity, and remedies for this situation were under consideration.

In general, the suite had fulfilled its major goals of low cost and convenience to patients and convenience to physicians. Physician acceptance was high, and a great deal of patient mail had been received praising the concept and the facility. The location of the facility also was well accepted by other patients and physicians. The physical connection to the hospital has been valuable in transferring patients who are not fully recovered by the end of the ambulatory surgery recovery-room hours. The transfers usually have been at the patient's request, rather than for purely medical reasons, because the patient did not feel well enough to cope with the home situation.

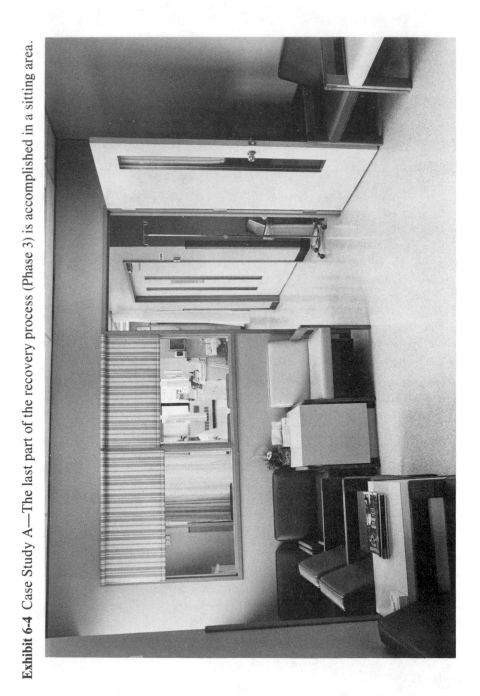

Exhibit 6-4 Case Study A—The last part of the recovery process (Phase 3) is accomplished in a sitting area.

Case Study B

The ambulatory surgical facility in Case Study B is owned by and fully integrated with a major medical center hospital. The medical center includes one of the largest integrated multispecialty clinics in the western United States. Ambulatory surgery is integrated with the hospital's preexisting inpatient surgery and with the emergency department that was built at the same time as the ambulatory surgical unit. This construction project included other hospital expansion and renovation (e.g., new main lobby, expanded dietary department, materials management, and critical care). The hospital has approximately three hundred beds.

Planning for this project began in late 1972. Since it was part of a hospital project, it came under certificate-of-need review. The project was completed, and the ambulatory surgical suite opened in 1976.

A fully integrated model type was selected for this facility. The selection was influenced by extreme land constraints on the campus, which provided few opportunities for a freestanding unit; concern for maximum staff efficiency; and the availability of recently acquired property near the existing inpatient surgical suite. Since ambulatory surgery service had been provided on a limited basis in the inpatient suite since the early 1960s, no problem in physician acceptance was anticipated. The physicians who would be the main users of the facility would have an all-weather connection to the unit through the hospital.

The location of the ambulatory surgical unit with the hospital's emergency room (which was not a major trauma facility) provided easily identifiable access and an immediately available automobile drop-off point to serve the ambulatory surgery.

Capacity and Size

This facility was designed to add five operating rooms to the inpatient suite, two of which (numbers 10 and 11 in Figure 6-2) were planned mainly for ambulatory surgery, though not on an exclusive basis. It was believed that each of these rooms could accommodate approximately six procedures per day, for a total capacity of approximately three thousand procedures per year.

Suite Arrangement

Entry to the ambulatory surgery is shared with the emergency department, which is directly served by an automobile drop-off point. The ambulatory surgery receptionist shares the emergency room reception desk (see Figure 6-2 and Exhibit 6-5). Patients wait for surgery in the same waiting

Figure 6-2 Floor Plan for Case Study B Ambulatory Surgical Facility

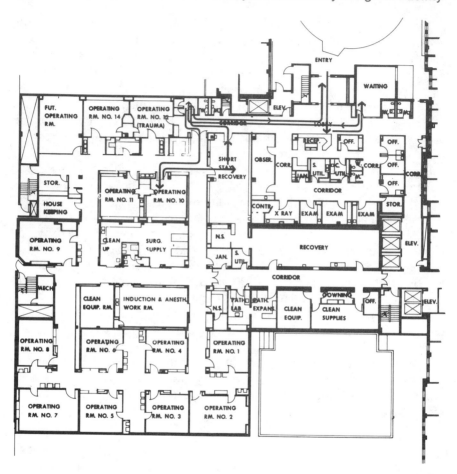

room as emergency patients (see Exhibit 6-6). They are summoned by the receptionist and taken to the dressing cubicles. From there, they are taken by a surgery assistant to the short-stay recovery room, where they receive instructions and climb onto a stretcher. Although this situation was not considered ideal, it was accepted as a way to achieve maximum flexibility in a very limited space used for preoperative preparation. From here, the patient is wheeled to the operating room, usually, but not always, to either room 10 or 11 (see Figure 6-2). Following the surgical procedure, the patient is wheeled back to the short-stay recovery room and held there until fully recovered.

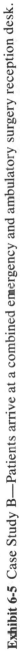

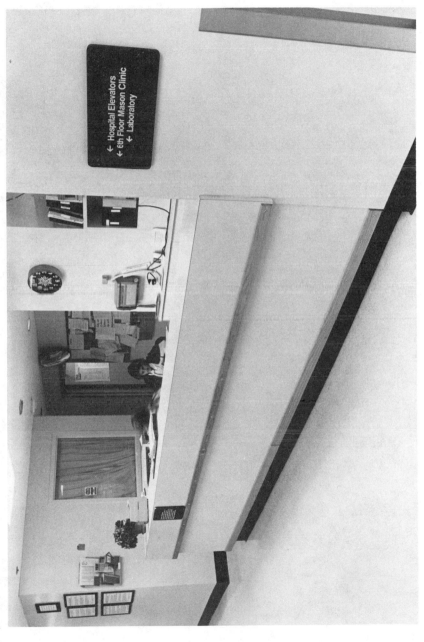

Exhibit 6-5 Case Study B—Patients arrive at a combined emergency and ambulatory surgery reception desk.

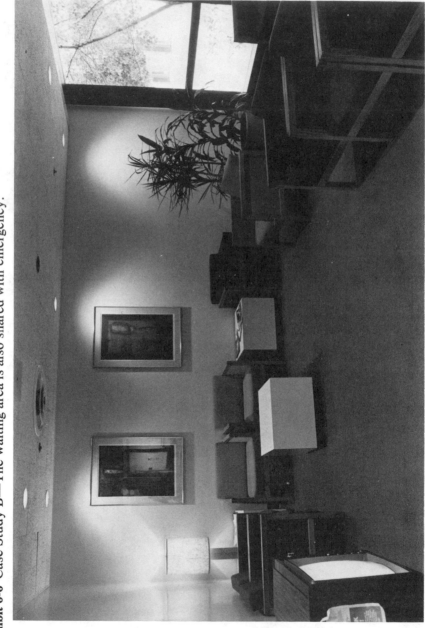

Exhibit 6-6 Case Study B—The waiting area is also shared with emergency.

The ambulatory surgical unit shares the material distribution system, anesthesia support area, and equipment storage facilities of the inpatient surgery suite. The recovery area is separate from but physically connected to the inpatient recovery area, which permits consolidation of recovery cases, if necessary, at the end of the day (see Exhibit 6-7). After recovery, the patient returns to the dressing area, dresses, and leaves, or is held in the waiting area until an escort arrives.

Staff dressing, locker, and lounge facilities are shared with the inpatient suite, and are located on a floor below the surgery suite, and are accessible to the dedicated stairway adjacent to the future operating room (see Figure 6-2).

Postoccupancy Evaluation

The performance of this suite was reviewed five years after it opened with the operating room supervisor and with the nurse in charge of ambulatory surgery. Although the suite was initially developed under very tight space constraints, due to the "landlocked" location, it has performed well. Significant lessons were learned from the five-year operating experience.

The combined use of the recovery area as a preoperatory preparation space has not been the problem originally anticipated, partly because operating room 12 is used by anesthesiologists for some of their preoperative interaction with the patient. Although still not considered ideal, it has been acceptable from the patients' standpoint and reasonably efficient for the staff.

The ability to use all operating rooms for either inpatient or ambulatory surgical cases may well have helped to avoid schedule problems for different types of procedures. The different peak load characteristics have complemented one another. Conflicts between the two surgical modes have been minimal. The likelihood of an ambulatory case being cancelled or postponed due to an emergency case has not been greater than for inpatient cases. The room sizes (approximately four hundred net square feet) are the same for both ambulatory surgery rooms and general inpatient surgery rooms, and are adequate for all inpatient procedures except those requiring extensive equipment (see Exhibit 6-8).

The use of the emergency waiting room for ambulatory surgery patients and their families has not created any significant problems. It is estimated that a peak of approximately six people wait for ambulatory surgery in this area at any one time. Occasionally, however, the waiting area becomes crowded due to a peak load during an emergency.

The mixing of postrecovery patient observation with other activities in the recovery area presents a significant problem. Plans are currently being

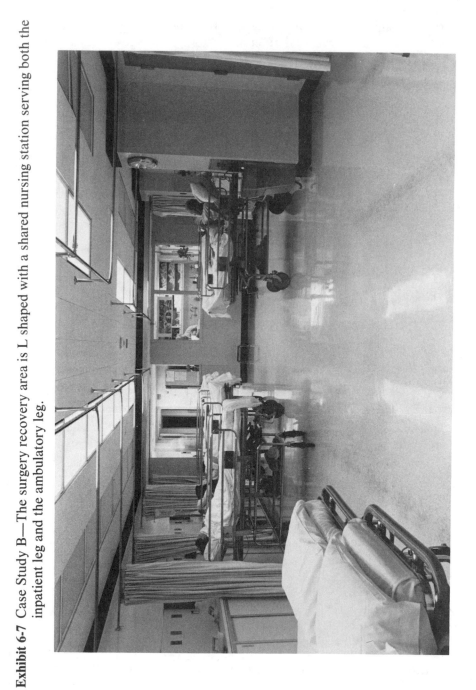

Exhibit 6-7 Case Study B—The surgery recovery area is L shaped with a shared nursing station serving both the inpatient leg and the ambulatory leg.

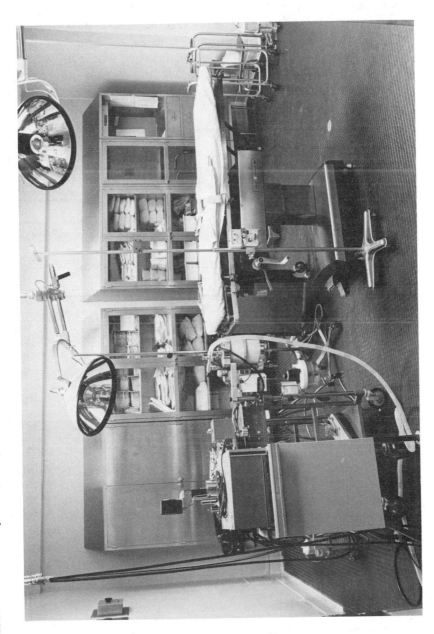

Exhibit 6-8 Case Study B—The operating room used for ambulatory cases is a standard general operating room.

made to create a separate postrecovery observation area for patients who are able to sit up. The recovery area now accommodates twelve patients. This capacity is considered tight on ambulatory surgery peak days (Thursdays and Fridays) when more than two operating rooms are used for ambulatory cases. This recovery area is also used by a pain clinic and a bronchoscopy suite that are located elsewhere in the hospital.

The actual ambulatory surgery workload had grown to over twenty-seven hundred cases by 1980, representing an increase of 19 to 28 percent of the total surgical caseload between 1975 and 1980.

One of the advantages of this ambulatory surgery model that was cited by the staff is the ability safely to attempt more complex cases on an ambulatory basis because of low risk to the patient if the mode of surgery must be changed during the procedure. Because more complex cases can be scheduled as ambulatory, 3 to 4 percent of scheduled ambulatory cases in this suite may end up as hospital admissions. The result is increased convenience and reduced cost of ambulatory surgery for a broader segment of surgical patients.

Although this suite was developed along quite different lines than the suite described in Case Study A, it too has fulfilled its major goals. The integration of the ambulatory surgery with the inpatient surgery produced a very efficient system from a staffing point of view. The facility also operated at significantly lower cost for ambulatory surgical cases than for inpatient cases, and it was convenient for physicians.

SUMMARY

This chapter has reviewed two existing ambulatory surgical facilities. Both units are hospital affiliated, but were developed along quite dissimilar lines. Both suites were developed with some physical constraints (aside from any capital cost constraints), which may have been considered desirable at the time. In Case Study A, the constraint was imposed by the limits of a single floor of a medical office building. In Case Study B, the constraint was imposed by the area available in the landlocked site.

Each suite was developed to respond to the specific needs of the sponsoring institution, to develop new service (Case Study A), and to continue an existing service in the most efficient way (Case Study B).

Five important lessons have been learned from the case study evaluations.

1. There is a trend toward more procedures requiring more extensive equipment in ambulatory surgery (e.g., arthroscopy, cataract repair).

It is therefore important to consider standard-size operating rooms that provide the flexibility to accommodate all unforeseen procedure types. The amount of equipment storage space should also be considered in light of this trend.

2. Once an ambulatory surgery recovery area is established (in a hospital or clinic setting), it may become a site for nonsurgical care programs because of the opportunity for short-term patient observation that it provides. This potential should be carefully analyzed during the planning and design stage in order to decide whether or not to provide for other programs, or to determine a reasonable strategy to accommodate them if the decision is later changed.

3. Although the patient cost structure for recovery time was not discussed in this chapter, it was considered an important issue at both case study sites, and a differentiation between inpatient and outpatient recovery costs in terms of hourly rates and time blocks charged was studied.

4. The workload capacity of a single ambulatory surgery operating room can approach six to eight cases per peak load day if a reasonable turnaround time is made available, and if the average times of procedures at these two facilities are reasonable guides. Due to patient scheduling preference, however, it seems unlikely that such a utilization rate is sustainable on a weekly basis, an overall average of four to five cases per day seems more realistic.

5. Some of the space reductions in these suites, which represented program compromises, proved to be workable (i.e., combined recovery and preoperatory preparation). These compromises, however, are still thought to be disadvantages and would not be repeated except under similar constraints.

There are a number of basic models for designing ambulatory surgical facilities. Each model has its place relative to the goals of a specific sponsor, and final implementation is influenced by the constraints and opportunities of the situation in which it is developed. To be successful, any design must accommodate the most universal goals of ambulatory surgery: lower cost to patients (as compared with inpatient surgery) and convenience for patients and physicians.

Chapter 7

Planning and Designing Ambulatory Surgical Facilities for Hospitals

Marlene J. Berkoff, AIA

With the rapidly increasing growth and popularity of hospital-sponsored ambulatory surgery services, more and more hospitals are faced with the need to build facilities to house ambulatory surgical centers, renovate existing areas for ambulatory surgeries, or create space in which ambulatory surgery programs can operate effectively.

To accomplish this task, the institutions must become knowledgeable about two major facets of creating a new facility, both of which are frequently unfamiliar. First, they must learn to understand and work with the architectural planning, design and construction process. To apply this process most advantageously to their particular projects, hospitals must acquire at least a basic comprehension of the activities and sequence of events that must occur; a knowledge of the available options and methods of approach; and an understanding of who participates in the process and why and when they participate. They must also develop a reasonable awareness of the background against which this process takes place. The current status of construction costs, codes, and regulations can significantly affect key decisions concerning the design and scope of a project, the time schedule, and the choice between building a new facility as opposed to renovating an old one or building a freestanding as opposed to an in-hospital unit.

Hospital management also must define a special functional product— the ambulatory surgical facility. Since ambulatory surgery is a relatively new service in most hospitals, with no tested historical precedent for planning or operation, this undertaking will not be a simple one. The success of the eventual ambulatory surgical unit, however, depends heavily

Adapted from *Journal of Ambulatory Care Management* 1981;3:35–51.

on the parent institution's ability to define clearly the scope and nature of the desired facility.

Before any firm decisions can be made about the size, cost, or design of the unit, and before any determination can be reached about its location or its potential for sharing hospital support services, questions must be discussed and resolved to the greatest degree possible concerning how the ambulatory surgical facility should function, who it should serve, when and how it should be utilized, what image it should convey, how it should interrelate with the hospital, and what its future should be.

There is no doubt that the planning, design, and construction process is a demanding, time-consuming, and frustrating task for hospital administrators, even if they have been involved in a construction project before. If they embark on an ambulatory surgical unit project, however, with a reasonable knowledge of the architectural process and a clearly defined concept of the functional goals they wish to achieve, they will have the maximum opportunity to create a facility that satisfies their requirements and is provided in a cost-effective manner.

EXTERNAL COST AND DESIGN DETERMINANTS

To a certain extent every construction project is governed by a number of external variables imposed by the economy and myriad regulatory bodies. Health care facilities are one of the most heavily regulated building types in the United States. In recent years they have also had to exercise extreme care to control costs. Although hospitals can do little about construction costs, codes, and regulations, it is essential that they be cognizant of these factors so that they can realistically plan facilities to be as cost-effective as possible and can meet applicable regulations without sacrificing functional or design concepts.

Construction Costs

We know we are living in a very inflationary economy. Construction costs, like all other costs, are continually escalating. The current annual rate of inflation for construction costs is approximately 10 percent, and no significant change is anticipated. Hospitals planning to develop new ambulatory surgical facilities or renovate old ones face strong pressures to move rapidly to beat inflation. In the current economic environment, any delay becomes costly.

Although the rate of inflation in construction costs applies to any facility being built, the actual range of costs depends largely on the building type and complexity. There are as yet no adequate data on construction costs for ambulatory surgical facilities, but a brief look at their characteristics demonstrates that they will not be very different from acute care hospitals.

An ambulatory surgical facility is a structure that houses a program for delivery of one-day surgical procedures. It is predicated on the assumption that scheduled operations will be performed; that these operations will require regional, local, or general anesthetic; and that patients will arrive and depart on the same day. Inpatient rooms are not provided for overnight stays. There are, however, operating rooms (ORs); recovery areas; examination rooms; toilet facilities; utility and service areas; perhaps laboratory, x-ray, business, and medical record areas; and staff and public space.

The ORs and recovery areas demand the same sophisticated mechanical and electrical support systems required of a hospital. Piped-in medical gases; emergency electrical power; isolated grounding systems; sophisticated communications systems; and special heating, cooling, and ventilating systems are required. Mechanical and electrical systems account for close to half the hospital construction costs; ambulatory surgical facilities have similar requirements for these expensive systems.

Ambulatory surgical facilities are not inexpensive to build. It can be reasonably anticipated that their cost will be similar to hospital construction costs, ranging considerably more than $100 per square foot in the early 1980s. Of course, when an ambulatory surgery program shares existing hospital operating suites or other services, the overall costs of construction are proportionately reduced.

Life-Cycle Cost Analysis

Initial construction costs loom large when a hospital is planning a new or renovated facility. Equally important, however, are the recurring operational costs of wages and salaries, maintenance, fuel, and utilities. These costs often constitute more than 80 percent of hospital expenses. Key planning and design decisions should be evalauted in terms of their potential impact on long-term operational costs and initial capital expenditures.

A two-story building may cost less to construct than a single-story building with equal space, because it requires less footings, foundation, and roof. The two-story configuration, however, may demand duplicate staff positions on two floors. A life-cycle cost analysis provides a systematic evaluation of such alternative solutions by considering all relevant economic consequences over the life cycle of the structure.[1] This analysis can help to determine the real cost impact of additional staff salaries versus initial construction cost savings, thereby providing the owners with a rational basis for making an informed design decision. Architects or consultants can help the hospital to apply a life-cycle cost approach, which is an especially valuable technique for assessing the implications of alternative locations or shared hospital services for ambulatory surgical units.

Value engineering deals with evaluating comparable costs for alternative design details or engineering systems, especially those related to energy use. These and other techniques of cost analysis are described by Robinson in a publication by the American Institute of Architects (AIA).[2] To plan, design, and construct a cost-effective facility, hospital management should be aware of these techniques and apply them early in the decision-making process. That is when such techniques can pay the greatest dividends in balancing initial capital expenditures, which are easily seen and understood, against recurring operational costs, which are more difficult to determine but which may have greater long-term impact.

Codes, Regulations, and Standards

A multitude of codes, regulations, and standards apply to health care facilities in general, and some now apply to ambulatory surgical facilities in particular. All these factors have considerable influence on cost and design. It is imperative that a hospital's architects or planners investigate all relevant codes and regulations prior to making any major design decisions. Although it is relatively easy to accommodate the provisions of most codes early in the architectural process, it later becomes exceedingly difficult and very expensive to modify plans to meet the requirements of an overlooked regulation. Compromise solutions and convoluted plans often result from this kind of oversight.

Probably the most ubiquitous standard applied to hospital construction is the National Fire Protection Association (NFPA) Life Safety Code 101.[3] The code has no legal authority, but it is cited as mandatory by numerous regulatory agencies. The Joint Commission on Accreditation of Hospitals (JCAH), Medicare and Medicaid, the Department of Health and Human Services (HHS), and many state and regional codes require compliance with the construction and fire safety standards of Code 101. Any ambulatory surgical facility—freestanding or in-hospital, new or renovated—that provides general anesthesia must meet the stringent health care occupancy requirements. The 1981 edition of Code 101 contains special sections (12-6 and 13-6) that directly apply to ambulatory surgical facilities.

Many other codes and regulations may apply to a specific ambulatory surgical facility. If federal funding is involved, the Department of Health, Education, and Welfare (now HHS) publication, entitled *Minimum Requirements of Construction and Equipment for Hospital and Medical Facilities*[4] may apply. Chapter 15 of the 1979 edition dictates minimum requirements for functional components, room sizes, mechanical systems, handicapped access, parking, and so on.

New standards have been formulated by the American National Standards Institute (ANSI) on accessibility for the physically handicapped. The NFPA publishes volumes of standards for mechanical, electrical, and plumbing systems. Major regional codes exist throughout the United States, as do many state and local building and health codes; the local codes are often more rigorous than the national ones. Many more regulations dealing with energy standards can be expected in the near future. Hospitals will have to continue working within this maze of codes and regulations, and they will have to comply with the most stringent standards of any applicable code.

PRELIMINARY PLANNING AND DESIGN PROCESS

The preliminary planning and design process for an ambulatory surgery should begin with several "pre-architecture" activities that establish the basic planning and design criteria and identify potential problem areas.

- Long-range goals and short-term functional objectives for the institution and its ambulatory surgery program must be established.
- Priorities among the goals and objectives must be identified as a rational basis for making the planning and design trade offs that always occur later in a project.
- Actual need and anticipated demand for ambulatory surgical services must be determined.
- Methods of practice and organization must be defined, both from a functional and an administrative perspective.
- All these criteria should be documented by the hospital, so that guidelines can be created and referred to throughout the long planning process, when original goals, priorities, and data are often obscured by the pressures of solving more immediate problems.
- Budget limitations and time constraints should be established to the greatest extent possible.
- Preliminary plans and concepts should be coordinated with the appropriate Health Systems Agency (HSA) if certificate-of-need (CON) approval is required.

Planning Organization

Establishing an effective in-house planning organization is one of the most important first steps in the planning process. The ambulatory surgery planning committee should include at least one representative of the surgical staff, as well as an anesthesiologist, a nursing director, and a hospital administrator familiar with the ambulatory surgery program and its relationship to other hospital services. This core group must be empowered to make decisions, and, if possible, its membership should remain consistent throughout the planning and design process.

Other departmental representatives should be included, as need dictates, to determine the necessary coordination with laboratory, radiology, central services, pharmacy, business and records, and physical plant services. Different strata of the user groups should be consulted to ensure a thorough understanding of how the ambulatory surgical unit will function at all levels, not just from the physicians' or supervisors' perspective.

A well-organized planning committee with an established decision-making structure can make the planning process far more effective for the hospital and the architectural team. Not only can a more accurate concept of the desired facility be generated, but also a great deal of very expensive time can be saved.

Planning and Design Professionals

The provider hospital will require the assistance of plannning and design professions for its ambulatory surgical facility. From the bewildering array of services available, the hospital must select those most appropriate and cost-effective for its particular needs.

At a minimum, the hospital will require architectural and engineering services. It may also need assistance in preliminary concept planning, program development, CON application, and determination of financial feasibility. Many of these services can be performed by a comprehensive architectural-engineering firm with experience in health facilities, but some will require specialized consultants. Services related to such project-delivery methods as construction management, contracting, and design-build may also be considered.

Hospital management should make every effort to learn about available professional services by talking with possible candidates, conferring with colleagues, and doing some homework. Publications are available from the AIA and the American Hospital Association (AHA) on selection of architects and methods of project delivery.[5-7]

THE ARCHITECTURAL PROCESS

The architectural process translates an initial need for an undefined functional space into a specific concept of defined scope, plan, and design, and ultimately into a three-dimensional physical structure that satisfies the original need within the constraints of the owner's schedule and budget. The traditional sequence of activities is:

- master planning
- programing
- schematic design
- design development and construction
- preparation of contract documents and bidding
- construction administration

Master Planning

Master planning defines broad concepts and creates guidelines for long-term growth and development of a hospital, its programs and services, and its physical facilities. If an ambulatory surgical unit is to be part of a hospital complex, the master plan should address its interrelationship with the other institutional facilities, present and future. Whether freestanding or in-hospital, on or off campus, the ambulatory surgical facility must be designed according to the master plan guidelines if it is to function as a well-integrated component of the hospital.

Programing

The architectural program is a narrative document that details the functional and space requirements for a particular facility. As described by Peña et al., architectural programing is "problem seeking."[8] The end product, the program document, is the problem statement. Peña defines five key steps in the programing process[8]:

- establish *goals*
- collect and analyze *facts*
- uncover and test *concepts*
- determine *needs*
- state the *problem*

This analytic approach to programing precludes premature attempts to arrive at a design solution before the problem is clearly stated. When planning an ambulatory surgical facility, this approach is especially valu-

able because the service is relatively new, there are no accepted proto-
types, and each case must be analyzed and defined in its own context.

Space Needs

The definition of room-by-room space needs is a pivotal component of
the architectural program; and it is more difficult to establish for ambulatory surgical services than for more stereotypical ones. The number, size,
and type of rooms depend on caseload and expected usage; mix of cases
to be performed; hours of operation; degree to which services will be
shared with the hospital; planned methods of operation; and desired flow
patterns for patients and staff.

It used to be an accepted rule of thumb, for example, that one OR could
handle about one thousand cases per year. Depending on the turnover
time of the cases and the hours during which the OR is used, however,
one dedicated ambulatory surgical OR may accommodate five to seven
cases per day and still terminate the outpatient schedule by 2:00 P.M.
Based on a five-day week, 1,300 to 1,820 cases per year could be performed
in a single OR.

If an OR is also used for inpatient cases, the number of ORs needed to
accommodate the ambulatory cases will be affected. It is therefore impossible to generalize. The number of ORs needed for an ambulatory surgery
must be determined according to the specific utilization patterns and sharing arrangements of the institution.

The method of operating an ambulatory surgical facility and the flow
patterns desired will also affect the room-by-room program. Some organizations want individual preoperative cubicles that can double as recovery
areas, eliminating the need for separate preparation and dressing spaces;
others prefer distinct areas for these functions. The space program must
reflect these different concepts. Flow diagrams, such as that shown in
Figure 7-1, can help planners to define how an institution's ambulatory
surgery should function—a necessary prelude to determining what rooms
to include.

Without an analysis of functional patterns, caseload, and mix, accurate
sizing of recovery space, holding space, preparation areas, or other support spaces is impossible. If an institution plans to provide a postanesthesia
recovery (PAR) area plus a second-stage recovery area, the PAR area will
require only one or two beds per OR. The number of spaces in the second-
stage recovery area can then be calculated, based on the estimated average
length of recovery time per patient and the rate of turnover expected in
the ORs.

It becomes apparent that space needs are largely interdependent with
the goals, facts, and concepts to be developed in the programing phase.

Figure 7-1 Ambulatory Surgery Patient Activity Flow Diagram

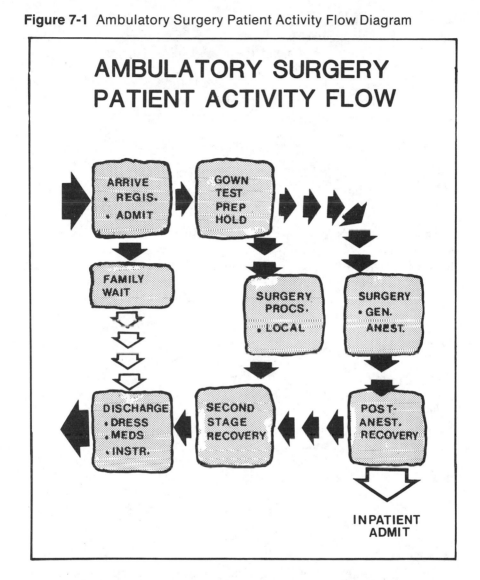

Although there are some "per-person" space relationships that can be used as general guidelines (such as 12 to 15 net square feet (NSF) for waiting areas, 75 to 100 NSF for recovery areas, and 80 to 100 NSF for office areas), these depend on the estimated number of people using the facility and the facility's method of operation.

The specific size of each room in an ambulatory surgical facility must be programed. According to the HEW minimum standards list, the minimum size of ambulatory surgical ORs is 250 NSF; and O'Donovan suggests that they can be smaller than inpatients units.[9] Other sources, such as Grubb and Ondov, recommend the more typical inpatient OR size of twenty-by-twenty feet, or 400 NSF, to provide flexibility for future utilization changes in technology or case mix.[10] In all instances, the size of each room depends on current and anticipated future use by patients and staff and on required equipment installations.

Functional Analysis

A thorough functional analysis of how the ambulatory surgery will work is perhaps the most critical element in designing an efficient unit. The circulation patterns for patients, staff, services, and supplies must be carefully examined in the context of a hospital or a freestanding setting. Flow diagrams provide one method of analysis. The proximity matrix, such as the example shown in Figure 7-2, provides a system for analyzing locational relationships and priorities for the components of the ambulatory surgical unit. These tools encourage the hospital planning committee and the architectural team to evolve and evaluate carefully the concepts that will serve as the basic guide for designing the facility.

Image

A major design determinant that is often overlooked is the image desired for an ambulatory surgical facility. The hospital administration may want the facility to appear as a separate, clearly identifiable unit that is isolated from the more institutional inpatient aspect of the building. Conversely, they may prefer to present the ambulatory surgical unit as an integral component of the hospital, emphasizing the clinical backup services and security of the parent institution. Each hospital must determine its own goals in the context of community setting, patient population, and competitive situation.

A carefully developed functional and architectural space program can be the most important determinant of a successful ambulatory surgical unit design. In the programing phase, few resources have been committed, and there is maximum opportunity for design flexibility. A clear and accurate problem statement of goals, concepts, and space needs provides the hospital and the architect with the necessary basis for developing a responsive solution to the real problem at hand.

Schematic Design

Schematic design is the first step in the problem solution. This architectural phase is the one during which functional organization and basic

Figure 7-2 Ambulatory Surgery Suite Proximity Matrix

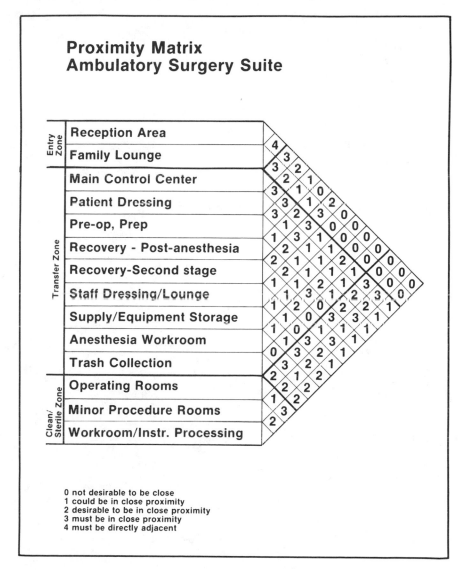

Proximity Matrix
Ambulatory Surgery Suite

Entry Zone
Reception Area
Family Lounge

Transfer Zone
Main Control Center
Patient Dressing
Pre-op, Prep
Recovery - Post-anesthesia
Recovery-Second stage
Staff Dressing/Lounge
Supply/Equipment Storage
Anesthesia Workroom
Trash Collection

Clean/Sterile Zone
Operating Rooms
Minor Procedure Rooms
Workroom/Instr. Processing

0 not desirable to be close
1 could be in close proximity
2 desirable to be in close proximity
3 must be in close proximity
4 must be directly adjacent

layouts are determined; design concepts of form, massing, and materials are developed; and major building and engineering systems are defined. Relationship diagrams, such as the one shown in Figure 7-3, help to resolve graphically the desired layout and circulation patterns, which are then

Figure 7-3 Ambulatory Surgery Functional Relationships

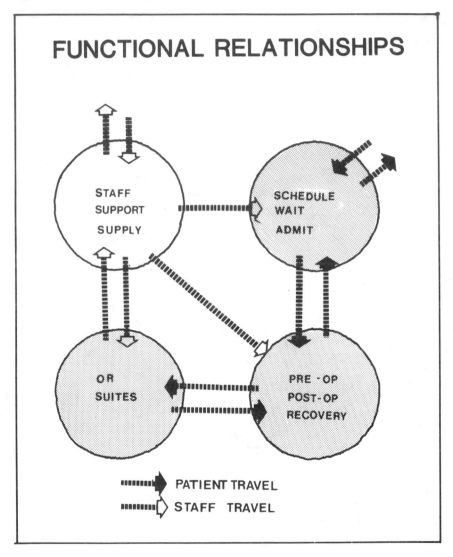

developed into preliminary floor plans. Sketch studies and models are also useful in determining and evaluating building form and image. The schematic development must be reviewed and approved by the ambulatory surgery planning committee before further refinement. At the end of this phase, a reasonably accurate cost estimate can and should be prepared, and the plans can be revised as necessary to meet budget restrictions.

Design Development and Construction

Once schematic plans are approved, all subsequent design development refines and further defines building form, plan, systems, and details. The ambulatory surgery planning committee and appropriate user representatives should work closely with the architectural team during this phase to fine tune the plans. Selections of cabinetry, built-ins, equipment, materials, colors, and design details must be made, reviewed, and approved. A final cost estimate should be prepared at the termination of this work.

Preparation of Contract Documents and Bidding

When the design development is complete, the architects and engineers prepare contract documents (plans and specifications) to convey all the requisite information to the contractors. These documents may then be released for competitive bidding, or contracts may be negotiated. The "fast-track" method, a variation of the traditional approach, speeds up this process by overlapping the design and construction phases. By determining such major design elements as the basic plan and structural system early in the process, partial contract documents can be prepared and construction can begin while other, more refined design details are still being resolved.

Construction Administration

The construction should be administered by an agent working in the owner's interest in order to ensure proper compliance with the contract documents and to assist in implementing any changes that occur. Depending on the method of project delivery, this agent may be the architect, construction manager, or some other field representative.

TWO MAJOR CHOICES

Two major choices often confront a hospital that is planning and designing an ambulatory surgical facility:

1. To build a new construction or to renovate existing space.
2. To build a freestanding facility or to locate the unit in or attached to the main hospital.

New Construction or Renovated Space

Hospitals face many pressures to renovate existing space, especially for ambulatory surgery. The ambulatory surgical facility is usually not large, and its requirements are frequently not well defined. It is often assumed that it can fit in almost anywhere. There are also cost savings to be realized by using existing space as opposed to creating new space. Several critical factors, however, should be evaluated before undertaking a major renovation project.

The useful life of the existing facility and the extent of remodeling required must be assessed. It is imperative to investigate the problems involved in bringing the existing facility into compliance with current codes. An architectural and engineering survey can make these determinations and permit the planners to decide if it is cost-effective even to consider using the existing space.

Designing the ambulatory surgery to fit into existing space can also pose problems. The existing building form or structural elements may prohibit a satisfactory space layout and seriously compromise the operational efficiency of the unit. Future flexibility and expansion may also be severely limited.

If the contemplated space is in the hospital, the planning team must evaluate the disruptive effects of the remodeling project. To avoid shutting down services during construction and to minimize disruption, the project may have to be carefully phased, increasing the time span and the costs of the work. Finally, it should be recognized that contractors frequently bid high on renovation work, especially in old structures, in order to cover the possible costs of dealing with unknown problems, such as unmarked mechanical chases or hidden structural obstacles.

Freestanding or In-Hospital Facilities

In addition to evaluating the comparative costs and benefits of building a new facility or renovating existing space, hospital management frequently needs to assess the trade offs between building a freestanding ambulatory surgical facility or an in-hospital or hospital-attached unit.

A freestanding facility, on or off the hospital campus, can be custom designed to provide an optimal space layout for the ambulatory surgery function without having to integrate with preexisting service locations and circulation systems. The desired image for the facility can be developed, and appropriate access routes and parking areas can be provided. Provisions for future expansion can be easily incorporated. The in-hospital unit frequently must compromise on all these elements.

The in-hospital ambulatory surgical facility, however, has the tremendous advantage of being able to share numerous hospital systems and services. The per-square-foot construction costs of a small, freestanding facility may be slightly less than comparable hospital building costs; but the in-hospital unit can almost always share existing conveyance systems, boiler plant, and all other major mechanical and electrical support systems. Even an ambulatory surgery addition to a hospital can generally be supported by small incremental increases in existing building systems, which a freestanding unit would have to duplicate at far greater cost.

The potential for sharing the medical and ancillary support services in a hospital setting is a mixed blessing. It is generally accepted that having the backup of an inpatient hospital is an asset in an emergency. It is also obvious that sharing existing services—such as central processing, medical records, laboratory, and radiology—eliminates duplication of space, equipment, and some staff. But the sharing arrangements usually create complex circulation patterns and complicate the organization of an efficient ambulatory surgical unit. The advantages and disadvantges of an in-hospital location must be carefully explored in each individual case. Three potential locations are usually considered: the emergency department, the outpatient department, and the inpatient operating suite.

Emergency Department

The main reason for developing an ambulatory surgical facility as an adjunct to the emergency department (ED) is that existing minor surgeries or procedure rooms are often underutilized and can double as outpatient ORs. The advantages of constant staffing and easy access are also frequently cited. The tense and sometimes chaotic environment of a busy ED, however, is in direct conflict with the calm and controlled atmosphere desired for an ambulatory surgical facility. The unpredictability of the ED constantly threatens the functional efficiency of the ambulatory surgery program by violating the basic planning premise that cases will be performed on schedule. The ED is thus a very undesirable location for an in-hospital ambulatory surgery.

Outpatient Department

An ambulatory surgery can be developed near other hospital outpatient areas. This location often permits the sharing of the reception, registration, waiting areas as well as some ancillary support functions, such as the outpatient laboratory and radiology. Parking and access may be easily developed in an area that already functions well for outpatient services. The main disadvantages of an outpatient area location are that new operating suites and recovery areas must usually be created, and staff and equipment duplications may occur. Initial development costs and long-term operating costs may be increased, although the benefits of sharing all the other hospital building and support services make this alternative less expensive than a completely separate, freestanding facility.

Inpatient Operating Suite

Probably the most cost-efficient in-hospital location is one that permits the sharing of the main hospital OR suite and PAR area (i.e., if adequate capacity exists or can be added at a modest increment). Surgical staff dressing areas, sterile supply, and anesthesia support can also be shared. The major problem with this option is that it is often very difficult to create distinct access routes and circulation patterns that separate the ambulatory patients and their friends and relatives from inpatient traffic.

As Figure 7-4 shows, successful, if not ideal, solutions to this problem are possible. This design features a new ambulatory surgery reception, preparation, and second-stage recovery area, with a separate elevator access, in a remodeled wing of an existing hospital. Being immediately adjacent to the main OR suite and PAR area permits maximum sharing and realizes significant cost savings.

Figure 7-5 depicts a solution that took advantage of an existing first-floor OR suite. A new addition created an ambulatory surgical unit, a new emergency unit, and a shared outpatient admissions area. Distinct outpatient and emergency entrances separate the traffic flow and still allow optimum sharing of new and existing facilities.

These examples demonstrate that less space and fewer functions need to be created for an in-hospital ambulatory surgery than for a freestanding unit, such as the one shown in Figure 7-6. Although this facility optimizes the flow patterns and expansion capabilities desired by the owner, all functional support and building systems had to be designed just to serve this structure.

DESIGN

In the competitive environment that confronts hospitals today, functional efficiency and cost effectiveness will not necessarily ensure a successful ambulatory surgical facility. Attention must also be devoted to creating an attractive setting that provides for patient comfort and convenience. Design concepts reflecting the image and identity the hospital wishes to convey should be developed from the earliest planning stages. A good design will be achieved not by simply applying wall graphics to an area once it is built, but by developing the size and scale of the spaces; the exposure to natural light; the circulation patterns; and the use of materials as integral components of the architectural process.

Figure 7-4 Ambulatory Surgery Located in Renovated Hospital Space

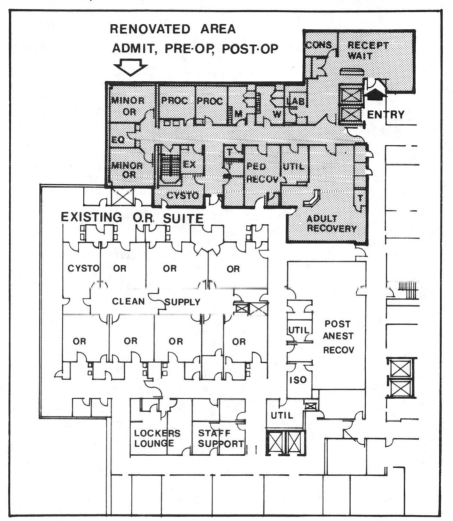

Patients electing to use an ambulatory surgical facility will be far more demanding of amenities—such as adequate waiting areas and toilet rooms, and privacy in treatment and consultation rooms—than their inpatient counterparts. An ambulatory surgical unit is predicated on same-day arrival and departure; thus, easy access, adequate parking, and clearly marked entry points and internal circulation routes also become critical to a suc-

Figure 7-5 Ambulatory Surgery Addition to an Existing Hospital

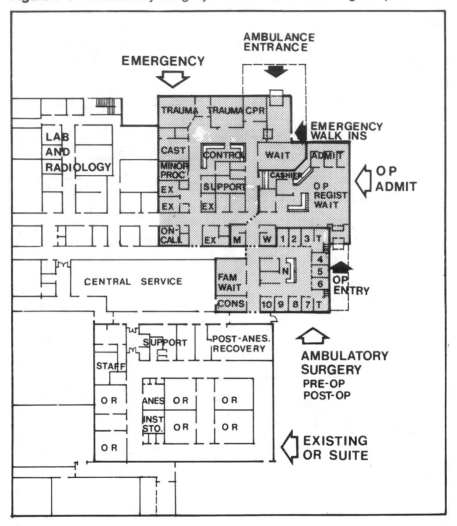

cessful design solution. Signage, carefully coordinated directional graphics, and orientation points become key elements in the design, especially in a hospital-based facility.

A sensitive use of building materials, room finishes, color, lighting, furniture, artwork, and plantings can contribute greatly to an atmosphere that promotes patient confidence and well-being and enhances staff satisfaction. Even in a busy hospital setting, carefully planned use of these

Figure 7-6 Freestanding Ambulatory Surgery Center

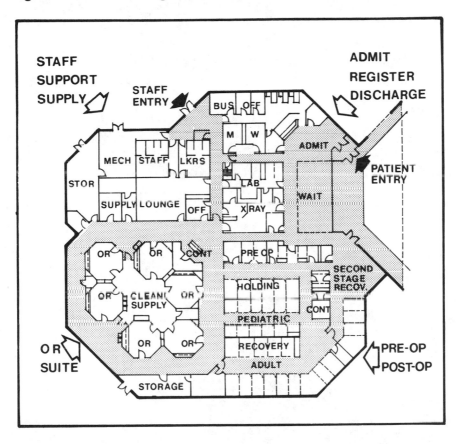

design elements can permit the creation of an attractive ambulatory surgical unit with an identifiable image. The planning and design of a successful ambulatory surgery ultimately depend on a joint effort by the parent hospital and the architectural team to establish accurate functional goals and design objectives; to thoroughly explore alternative options; and to develop the solution that best meets the program criteria in a cost-effective manner.

REFERENCES

1. American Institute of Architects: *Life Cycle Cost Analysis: A Guide for Architects.* Washington, DC, American Institute of Architects, 1977.

Chapter 8

Presbyterian Hospital of Dallas: An Ambulatory Surgery Program

Douglas D. Hawthorne, M.S.

In February 1972 in the Austin, Texas, *American Statesman* a headline read: "Woman Has Surgery and Returns Home the Same Day." At that time it was unique for a patient to go to the hospital, have surgery, and return home the same day. Today this pattern has become an integral part of the health care delivery in U.S. hospitals.

Ambulatory surgery has existed for more than 100 years, but it was not until new types of anesthesia agents were improved that faster recovery of patients was possible. Because of this development, "one-day-stay" programs began to develop. Ambulatory surgery is known under many terms, such as in-and-out surgery, come-and-go surgery, day surgery, one-day surgery, short-stay surgery, and most recently ambulatory surgery. No matter what term is used, the concept means that the patient has a surgical procedure and goes home the same day, thus eliminating the traditional hospital admission, overnight hospitalization, and discharge.

Presbyterian Hospital of Dallas, Texas, initiated an ambulatory surgery program in 1970 in response to a high patient census, which was causing long delays for elective surgical procedures. To expedite implementation, the program was integrated into existing facilities and services. In the past ten years, Presbyterian Hospital has provided ambulatory surgery to more than forty thousand patients.

THE INTEGRATED PROGRAM

Typical full-service, acute-care community hospitals have inherent resources to provide most levels of medical service. In many instances these resources are not fully utilized on a 24-hour-a-day basis. Since these

Adapted from *Journal of Ambulatory Care Management* 1981;3:53–60.

resources were already available, it was decided early at Presbyterian Hospital to provide an ambulatory surgery program within the existing structure.

In the early 1970s, it was not known how such a program would work as an alternative to conventional overnight surgery, but in reviewing its potential, it appeared that it would allow better overall utilization of inpatient beds and better service to more patients.

An experimental program was initiated whereby existing space for recovery beds was used and day surgery procedures were performed in the existing operating rooms. Some additional staff were needed, but no facility modifications were required. Construction of a new operating room would have cost approximately forty thousand dollars and required additional staff, backup resources, and a major duplication of facilities and services that were already available. Although the addition of day-surgery cases to the existing surgical load necessitated more staff, it allowed for better overall utilization of the operating room and recovery room space.

When the program was integrated into the existing facilities, it was found that staff members in all areas could adjust relatively easily to one-day-stay patients; that the items needed to carry through on one-day surgery were available in the operating room, recovery room, and anesthesia areas; and that patients were in and out of the operating room-recovery room area before the major cases began.

The decision to integrate required hospital personnel to modify their routine methods. Ambulatory surgery must be convenient and comprehensive because of the short duration of the patient's stay, which is not typical of conventional inpatient admissions. If the program was to be successful, staff had to be attuned to the purposes behind the ambulatory surgery program. To help achieve this, an in-service education and orientation process took place for all hospital personnel involved with the day-surgery program.

PROGRAM ACCOUNTABILITY

Because the program was to be integrated into a traditional hospital setting, it was necessary to establish goals and objectives for management, nursing, and medical staff, and to establish accountability for meeting those goals and objectives.

Management

Management desired from the start to free inpatient surgical beds for the more sophisticated, time-consuming surgical cases and eliminate long waiting periods for elective surgical procedures. In essence, these became the goals of the program.

Management soon discovered that substantial cost savings were accruing to patients and third party payers as a result of the program. The elimination of one- and two-night stays in the hospital and of certain ancillary charges reduced overall hospital cost. It also increased patient census by cutting down waiting periods and improved utilization of inpatient surgical beds.

The initial cost of the program was minimal because it was integrated into existing facilities; therefore, management was successful in accomplishing the original objectives of the program. They also helped create high patient and physician satisfaction levels. Patients' satisfaction was tested by means of telephone surveys. The items that received consistent, positive responses were: (1) the convenience of getting in and out of the hospital; (2) the opportunity to return home on the day of surgery and to be assisted in the recovery process by relatives; (3) to return to a job or to school soon after surgery; and (4) the reduced cost of this hospitalization program. Physician satisfaction was tested by verbal inquiry of the major users. The items of greatest satisfaction to the physican were: (1) convenience of a single visit to one facility; (2) availability of all resources necessary for backup and emergency situations; and (3) ability to admit more patients to the hospital and reduce waiting time.

Management accountability was controlled by periodically reviewing program functioning. The setup of the facility was a control factor (see Figure 8-1). The patient bedroom area for the ambulatory surgery program was a totally integrated area but was within the mainstream of the hospital. These independent beds were constructed exclusively for one-day-stay patients and had the necessary preadmission workup area, family room, dietary facilities, medication area, nursing station, and supply areas. The unit was established as a separate cost center and directly controlled as a typical nursing unit. The Day Surgery Unit was responsible for its own staff and the development of the policies and procedures for its operation. Hospital administration controlled the unit through its Nursing Service and made it accountable through budget control.

Nursing

The Nursing Service was expected to create an environment different from that of the typical inpatient nursing unit. Staff were selected based on their ability to give comprehensive, relaxed, and pleasant service to one-day-stay patients. Nursing accountability was monitored through their nursing documents, which were used for periodic review. The integration

Figure 8-1 Twenty-bed day surgery unit, Presbyterian Hospital

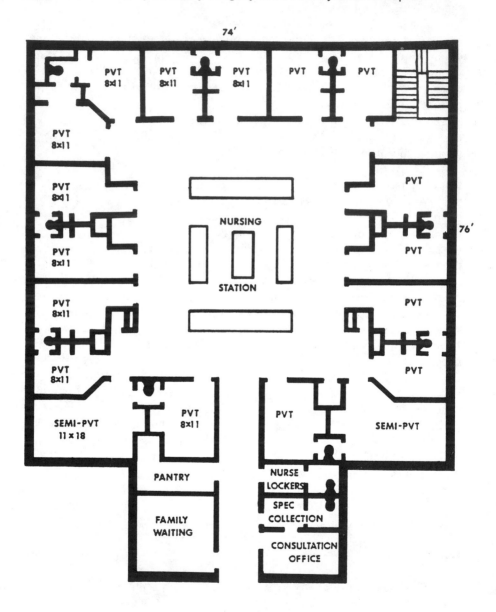

of the program into the hospital made accountability of the Nursing Service easier, because in the operating room and recovery room the same nurses were associated with both day-surgery patients and conventional surgical patients.

Medical Staff

Medical staff accountability lies with the members of the Operating Room Committee of the medical staff. The committee determines what cases are appropriate for a day-surgery program and initiates certain procedures that set the program apart from the conventional surgery program. Such procedures include:

- setting up day-surgery procedures to be performed in sixteen of the eighteen operating rooms at the start of each day (7:30 A.M.);
- block booking to allow physicians to perform day-surgery cases one right after the other;
- establishing mandatory cutoff times for one-day-stay patients of 12:00 P.M. (so that adequate recovery time would be available prior to the closing of the unit at 6:00 P.M. daily);
- writing physician discharge orders, which necessitated the anesthesiologist or surgeon to see patients prior to patients' discharge (telephone orders were unacceptable because it was difficult to judge the condition of patients with such a short time in the hospital, and it was necessary for the anesthesiologist or surgeon to examine patients prior to their leaving the unit.)

As partial control of medical staff accountability, the program is reviewed by the Utilization Review and Quality Assurance Program of the hospital.

CHARGING AND REIMBURSEMENT

Because in the early 1970s day surgery was a new concept, Presbyterian Hospital's management was required to solicit the support of the major insurance carriers for the new program. The carriers indicated they would support the program and reimburse for the service only on an inpatient basis.

In most cases in the early 1970s, insurance policies did not have outpatient coverage and therefore could not reimburse for the program on an outpatient basis. Today this has changed; most of the insurance policies now provide for 100 percent coverage of ambulatory surgery. The distribution of reimbursement for the program currently is as follows:

- Blue Cross and Blue Shield = 24 percent
- other private third party payers = 54 percent
- Medicare and Medicaid = 2 percent
- self pay = 19 percent
- other = 1 percent

Charges to the patient were developed as routine charges that were applicable to the inpatient. Comparative analysis shows that in 1972 in the areas of operating room, recovery room, and anesthesia, charges for day-surgery patients were proportionate to charges for inpatients having the same procedure. The cost to the hospital for providing these services was the same for both patients, and was perhaps much lower than what it might have been if an all-new facility had been built to house the program. Charges to patients were reduced by eliminating overnight stays and—as was discovered after some historical data on the program was compiled—by decreasing the use of many of the support services, such as central service, pharmacy, laboratory, and x-ray. It was discovered by staff physicians that one-day-stay patients needed fewer supply and medication items, which reduced their charges. An all-inclusive charge per patient by surgical procedure has been instituted. This practice eliminates the necessity of centralizing all charges, doing several billings, and maintaining excessive financial records on each patient.

TYPES OF PROCEDURES

When the program began it was necessary to review Professional Activities Study (PAS) statistics to determine typical one- and two-night stays in the hospital as a result of surgery. A list was developed and distributed to a medical-staff advisory group, who added additional cases they thought applicable. The initial list included twenty procedures; today it includes over 100, of which the most frequently performed are:

- dilatation and curettage
- tonsillectomy and adenoidectomy
- cystogram and pyelogram
- myringotomy
- laryngoscopy

- dental extraction
- breast biopsy
- bilateral ocular-muscle procedure
- ganglionectomies
- scar revision
- miscellaneous procedures (excisions, circumcisions, cast changes, tubal ligation)

These procedures represent approximately 66 percent of all cases performed.

In order for a new procedure to be approved for day surgery, it must go before the Operating Room Committee of the medical staff. They review the case and determine its applicability; if approved, the procedure is added to the existing list. It is significant that 96 percent of the cases for the ambulatory surgery program at Presbyterian Hospital are performed under general anesthesia. This fact classifies them as typical hospital procedures and distinguishes them from the typical procedures performed in a physician's office (treatment of ingrown toenails, removal of certain skin lesions, etc.). As indicated, the procedures approved for day surgery are those that have traditionally been performed on a conventional basis; therefore, from a technique standpoint in the operating room-recovery room area, there is no change. Nursing personnel are familiar with these day-surgery cases as well as the more extensive cases, which creates the cost-saving advantage of eliminating the duplication of personnel expense.

A change that is occurring in the one-day-stay program is the inclusion of diagnostic procedures. Certain diagnostic procedures, such as heart catheterization and angiography, which have traditionally required overnight stays in the hospital, can now be performed on a one-day-stay basis. Again, the advantage is the fact that all these diagnostic laboratories are available in the hospital.

It is anticipated that additional ways of using the one-day-stay program will be developed, not only for surgical procedures, but for diagnostic procedures as well.

PATIENT FLOW PROCESS

The most important aspect of integrating an ambulatory surgery program into the hospital setting is to prevent one-day-stay patients from getting tangled in the traditional red tape of the hospital. Presbyterian Hospital has accomplished this.

Patients come to the hospital the day before their scheduled surgery, going directly to the admitting office between the hours of 9:00 A.M. and 12:00 P.M. Directing patients to come to the admitting office during this time avoids getting them involved in typical hospital admissions, which occur between 1:00 and 5:00 P.M. Day-surgery patients sign the paperwork that has been previously acquired through preadmission telephoning, and are escorted to the Day Surgery Unit. The nurse in the Day Surgery Unit obtains information from the patients for use by the anesthesiologist, including vital signs, allergies, and a brief health history. Specimens are then drawn and taken to the laboratory for processing.

The patients are given an opportunity to see the room they will be occupying the next day and are given an overall description of the surgical procedures. This familiarization session helps set the patients at ease. The patients then return home and come back to the Day Surgery Unit the next morning.

The patients are transported from a private room in the unit to the main operating room, where the surgical procedure is performed. Following the procedure (the average length of time for a procedure is sixty-five minutes) the patients go directly to the main recovery room area (the average length of stay is fifty-five minutes). The patients are then transported back to the private room in the Day Surgery Unit. The flow is easy and works within the existing transportation system for conventional surgical patients.

Most patients remain in the Day Surgery Unit 3½ to 4 hours, after which they are discharged. The care they receive during recovery is comprehensive. Registered nurses carry out physicians' orders and constantly observe and review the patient's condition. Light meal service and television are available, and all rooms have adequate seating for family and friends. In essence, day-surgery patients receive the same care as conventional patients.

Patients who develop complications in the operating room bypass the Day Surgery Unit after the procedure and go directly to a conventional surgical bed. Other patients whose condition has been determined by staff in the Day Surgery Unit to require further observation are transferred directly from the unit to a conventional bed for an overnight stay.

UTILIZATION STATISTICS

Presbyterian Hospital completed its fifteenth year of operation in May 1981. Since its inception, the number of hospital admissions has continued to grow. During the past five years total hospital admissions rose as follows: 1975–76: 27,884; 1976–77: 28,604; 1977–78: 29,495; 1978–79: 31,335; 1979–80: 33,567; 1980–81: 36,482. Innovative thinking by management and medical staff has allowed new programs to be developed that have helped increase patient activity and improve services.

Day Surgery Unit statistics also reflect annual increases, with a positive effect on the overall utilization of the operating room and recovery room area. By allowing the day-surgery program to be part of the overall hospital program, growth has been stimulated in other surgical services by virtue of freeing the conventional surgical bed.

PROGRAM SUCCESS

Initiation of the ambulatory surgery program at Presbyterian Hospital was a stopgap measure. With high occupancy and long waiting times for surgical procedures, there had to be an alternative that would allow the institution to continue to provide service but achieve better overall utilization of resources. At the time, little thought was given as to whether the program was appropriate for the long-range hospital mission. Not long after the program began, however, it became clear that the purpose and outcome of the program coincided directly with those of the hospital. The ambulatory surgery program met the hospital's objective of providing service to patients at a level consistent with patients' needs and at a price proportionate to that level of care. An additional bonus was the resulting increased satisfaction among health care personnel involved in the program.

Chapter 9

Crouse-Irving Memorial Hospital Freestanding Surgery Center Exceeds Expectations

James W. Maher

The one-day surgery center operated for more than four years by Crouse-Irving Memorial Hospital in Syracuse, New York, is an unqualifed success. Patients are saving time and money. Physicians are assured that the procedures they schedule will not be bumped or canceled by emergencies. Center staff personnel seem to enjoy working in a carefully controlled and relatively stress-free environment in which the absence of acute cases ensures patient care that is personal and positive.

The hospital's board of trustees and administration also consider the center highly successful for the following reasons:

- It is exceeding projected expectations in terms of patient and physician acceptance.

- It has not adversely affected the use of the hospital's fourteen operating rooms (ORs) or the hospital's daily census as some had feared it would.

- It functioned on a break-even basis for 2½ years using the originally established low patient charges, and, when the initial rates were increased in mid-1980, it became a money-making asset for the hospital.

To understand how the surgery center came into being and why it functions so well, it is necessary to view its evolution in light of changes at Crouse-Irving Memorial Hospital during the 1960s and 1970s.

Adapted from *Journal of Ambulatory Care Management* 1981;3:61–73.

EVOLUTION

Initial Merger

The physical merger of Crouse-Irving Hospital and Syracuse Memorial Hospital was completed in 1968, the first official year of existence for Crouse-Irving Memorial. Although the two facilities were located across the street from each other, there were much broader distances extant in the philosophical and practical ways the two hospitals functioned. The processes required to successfully bridge these gaps and effect an efficient new entity—the largest acute-care general hospital in the fourteen-county central New York region—were lengthy, complex, and painful at times. But they produced an unexpected benefit that has meant much to the growth of the hospital and its services.

That benefit can best be summarized as a "can-do" attitude. The board members, administrators, staff, and physicians who suffered through the difficulties enjoyed the accomplishments that resulted from the merger experience and adopted the attitude that they could do anything required to maintain and expand the care capabilities of their new hospital.

This collective positive attitude provided impetus throughout the remainder of the 1970s for the construction of a new eight-story Irving unit, which is connected to the Memorial unit. This new building contains the Emergency and Radiology departments; fourteen ORs and related facilities; the coronary, intensive, and progressive acute-care units; and three medical-surgical floors of seventy-six beds each.

Other major advances included construction of an addition to the old Syracuse Memorial Hospital structure to house the first childbirth center in central New York. This facility was designed expressly to accommodate traditional birth, scheduled and emergency Caesarean sections, and birthing room deliveries with or without a "coach" in attendance.

A 680-car parking garage and the Physicians Office Building were constructed across the street from the Crouse-Irving and Syracuse Memorial units and connected to them by a tunnel. The old Crouse-Irving Hospital was renovated to accommodate the hospital's school of nursing and a hostel residence for ambulatory patients and the families of out-of-town inpatients.

The surgery center, along with new advance registration and testing facilities, was planned for and built into the Physicians Office Building. But the decision to include an ambulatory surgical facility of this type was based on four years of prior in-hospital experience.

In-and-Out Unit

A six-bed "in-and-out" surgery unit was opened in the former Crouse-Irving Hospital in 1962. By 1970 the unit had grown to nineteen beds. For the most part, patients were admitted, had surgery in one of the hospital's regular operating rooms, went from recovery to the in-and-out unit, and were discharged the same day. Constant growth in size and use of this original unit prompted the decision in 1973 to develop a freestanding surgical center.

Internal research conducted by the administration brought to light the fact that as much as 25 percent of the typical annual surgical caseload could be handled in the kind of freestanding facility envisioned. Other in-house studies showed that a separate surgery center with a separate cost center would allow center charges to be minimized while eliminating the need for the center to comply with certain regulatory and procedural requirements imposed on the hospital. A subsidiary corporation was formed, which became the general partner in the Physicians Office Building venture.

Construction and Layout

The surgery center was built to specifications in the ten thousand square feet of space that constituted the seventh floor of the eight-story structure. The facility was then leased to the hospital under a turnkey arrangement. Construction cost was nine hundred thousand dollars, with a payback program of approximately twenty-one thousand dollars per month in rent for fifteen years.

As Figure 9-1 shows, the center layout is designed around a four-OR nursing station core. About seventy-five procedures are performed in these four ORs, the eye laser treatment room, and the minisurgery room. (A complete list of procedures is provided in Table 9-1.) Operations that take place in minisurgery require no recovery time, and local anesthesia is administered by the patient's physican (see Table 9-2.)

The majority of the procedures, however, involve one of the ORs and the administration of general anesthesia by an anesthesiologist or local anesthesia by a physician, monitored by an anesthesiologist.

TYPICAL PROCEDURE

Patients must report to the Advance Registration and Testing Center on the first floor of the Physicians Office Building two or three days before

Figure 9-1 Surgery Center Floor Plan

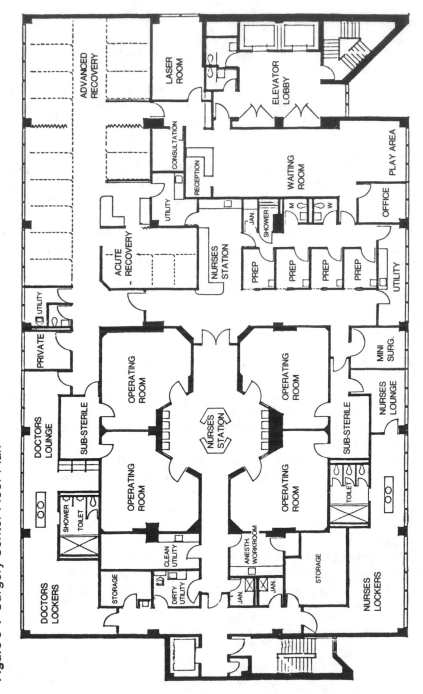

Table 9-1 Procedures Done in Surgery Center

Cardiopulmonary
Bronchoscopy
Replace Batteries, Pacemaker
Esophageal Dilatation

Dental
Multiple Fillings
Total Extraction
Removal of Impacted Teeth

ENT
Tonsillectomy and Adenoidectomy
Tonsillectomy and Adenoidectomy with
   Myringotomy
Adenoidectomy
Adenoidectomy with Myringotomy
Tonsillectomy
Tonsillectomy with Myringotomy
Myringotomy
Excision of Lesions
Laryngoscopy
Closed Reduction Nasal Fracture
Pharyngoscopy
Nasal Polypectomy
Submucous Resection
Rhinoplasty

General Surgery
Inguinal Herniorrhaphy
Vasectomy
Decompression of Median Nerve
Umbilical Herniorrhaphy
Excision of Ingrown Toenail
Breast Biopsy
Hydrocelectomy
Excision of Ganglion Cyst
Excision of Hypoglossal Duct Cyst
Circumcision
Excision of Lesions
Excision of Pilonidal Cyst
Repair Tendon
Node Biopsies

Gynecology
Exam under Anesthesia (EUA), Dilata-
   tion and Currettage (D & C)
D & C with Diagnostic Laparoscopy
   (Open, Closed)
D & C with Tubal Coagulation

D & C, Suction Curettage
Tubal Coagulation
Cystoscopy
Sigmoidoscopy
Minilaparotomy
Bartholin Cysts
Fulguration Condylomata

Neurosurgery
Decompression of Median Nerve

Ophthalmology
Recession Resection Eye Muscles
Exam Under Anesthesia (EUA) Bilateral
   Eyes
Probing of Tear Duct
Mebelene Sling to Frontalis Muscle
Excision of Lesion Eyelids
Incision and Biopsy, Chalazion
Fasanella Procedure, Lid
Cryotherapy
Cataract Extraction, with or without Lens
   Implant
Iridectomy

Orthopedics
Plastic Repairs
Excision and Removal of Foreign Body
Decompression of Median Nerve
Excision, Inclusion of Cyst Stump
Syndactylization of Toes
Release Tupuytrens Contracture Hand
Release Trigger Thumb
Z Plasty
Release Dequervains Hand
Excision of Ganglion
Remove plates, screws
Flexor tendon sheath release
Excision of Lesion
Open Reduction Fracture
Bunionectomy
Excision of Exostosis
Diagnostic Arthroscopy
Operative Arthroscopy

Pediatrics
Umbilical Herniorrhaphy
Inguinal Herniorrhaphy
Orchidopexy

Table 9-1 continued

Circumcision	Repair Tendon
Excision of Lesions	Blepharoplasty
Meatotomy	Rhytidectomy
Urethral Dilatation	Mammoplasty
Cystoscopy	Skin Grafts

Plastic	*Urology*
Excision of Ganglion	Cystoscopy
Fasciectomy	Biopsy Fulguration of Bladder Tumor
Release Trigger Fingers	Irrigation of Bladder
Revision of Scars	Biopsies
Repair Laceration	Circumcision
Release Contracture	

Additional Procedures
Blood Transfusions
Dermatology Laser Treatment for Hemangiomas, Port Wine Stains, Spider Veins, Telangiectasia
Eye Laser Treatment for Diabetic Retinopathy, Vein Obstructions, Glaucoma, Neovascularizations

Table 9-2 Surgery Center Minisurgery Procedures

Aspiration of Breast Lumps	Excision of Lipomas
Bilateral Vasectomy	Excision of Sinus Track
Biopsy of Liver	Excision of Tattoos
Biopsy of Temporal Artery	I & D, Chalazion
Biopsy of Muscle	I & D, Hematoma
Biopsy of Vulva	Marsupialization of Cyst
Blepharoplasty	Nerve Block
Bone Marrow Aspiration	Nerve Repair
Breast Implants	Paracentesis
Circumcision	Pinch Skin Grafts
Cryotherapy	Release Tendon Sheath Wrist
Debridement of Wounds	Release Trigger Finger
Diagnostic Lumbar Puncture	Removal of K Wires and/or Pins
Diathermy of Eyes	Removal of Plantar Warts
Excision of Condylomata and Fulguration	Removal of Toenail and/or Fingernail
	Repair Ectropion and Entropion
Excision of Cysts	Skin Flaps
Excision of Ganglions	Thoracentesis
Excision of Lesions	Z Plasty

scheduled surgery. Physicians schedule surgery center cases through the hospital's registrar's office but are also required to estimate the time required for the procedure.

Control Criteria

The most important control criterion for efficient and economical use of the center is that *no operations requiring more than one hour in the OR are scheduled in the center,* and the sixty-minute limitation includes all preparative and postoperative activities that must take place in that room.

Other criteria are that the patient must

- require elective surgery under general or local anesthesia;
- be in good general health; and
- be able to be safely discharged no later than 5:00 P.M. the same day.

Emergencies are excluded from the program. Patients with controlled systemic disorders may be eligible if an anesthesiologist is consulted and approves.

Necessary Information

After the physician has made the initial contact, the registrar's office mails a letter of explanation, brochure, form for required financial information, and appointed time for pretesting. Pretesting includes complete blood cell count (CBC) and urinalysis for all patients; these costs are included in the hospital's base charge for the surgery. A chemical profile is required for patients over thirteen years, and an electrocardiogram and chest x-ray are required for those over forty years who are to receive general anesthesia. Hospital costs for these procedures are reflected as extra charges.

In addition to registration and testing, patients are required to pay the hospital charges during prestesting or to supply proof of a valid reimbursement source. Patients also visit the surgery center to view an audio-visual presentation that explains what will take place the day of the operation. There are two presentations: one is designed for and shown only to patients thirteen years and under; the other is for those over thirteen. The interview with the anesthesiologist usually takes place at this time.

Patients are instructed to be at the surgery center two hours before their procedure is scheduled to be performed. Some of this time is needed to prepare for surgery, but the primary reason for early arrival is to maintain the tight schedule on which the center literally and figuratively operates.

The following data must also be at the surgery center by this time:

- history and physical
- preoperative orders
- required laboratory work
- OR permit that has been secured and witnessed by physician

Optimal Care

Patients and those accompanying them wait in a bright, spacious, comfortable area that includes reading materials, coffee, and a variety of quiet diversions for children. The preparation rooms are only a few steps away.

Usually, one nurse is assigned as liaison on each case; the nurse meets the patient and any family or friends in attendance; takes the patient into the preparation room; and stays with the patient during the advanced recovery period, when the patient is allowed family visitors. As Figure 9-1 shows, physicians and staff members are never far from any patient or equipment, yet adequate private space is also provided and comfortably appointed for physicians and nurses.

EFFICIENCY FACTOR

Everything and everyone involved with the surgery center is geared to a highly efficient workday (i.e., every weekday) without giving patients the feeling that they are involved in a tightly controlled process. This atmosphere is created through careful planning and execution. Three areas have already surfaced: spatial relations within the facility; strict criteria for patients and physicians; and preplanning that includes registration, testing, patient orientation, and financial arrangements.

Another area of efficiency is paper work. Only three basic 8½- by 11-inch forms are involved:

- A patient identification form (one page) filled out by the physician. One side contains medical history; physical examination information; physician's orders; and space for progress reports, OR and discharge notes, nurses' signatures, and sign offs by the attending physician and anesthesiologist. The operative and anesthetic consent form is on the other side.
- An OR-recovery room checklist and report form (one page) for use during the procedure and recovery. This side serves as the patient's

"chart." The reverse side contains the medical history information supplied by the patient plus input from the testing center, the interviewing anesthetist, and the admitting nurse.

- A surgery center procedure record (one page with three carbon sets), which provides all information usually required for medical record billing and accounting purposes.

Two types of postoperative instruction forms are also available. Physicians using the facility regularly are supplied with mimeographed forms with their instructions for specific procedures. All these physicians need do is add special instructions or comments, if any, and sign the form. The other type is a prepared form that requires the physician to fill in relevant areas, including diet, medication, and incision care.

ORGANIZED STRUCTURE

The surgery center averages twenty-eight operations a day and is open eight hours every weekday, from 7:00 A.M. to 5:00 P.M. First procedures take place at 8:00 A.M., and the last procedures requiring general anesthesia are scheduled no later than 1:15 P.M.

Figure 9-2 shows the administrative and organizational structure of the facility. Flexible staffing shifts allow for a minimum personnel complement. Tight scheduling of procedures provides maximum usage of the facility within the time frame established. And, because patients are required to arrive two hours before the operation, scheduled procedures can be juggled when an emergency prevents a physician or a patient from honoring the commitment.

As Figure 9-2 indicates, there is no medical director for the surgery center. Instead, there is a surgery center committee consisting of physician representatives from the hospital's specialty surgery services and the anesthesiology department; the center director and head nurses; and a vice-president who represents the hospital administration.

This committee has been instrumental in effecting good relations between the medical staff and the facility. Physician rules are agreed on in advance by the committee. Should a physician violate a rule, the committee takes the responsibility of communicating the problem to the physician and working out a solution. Conversely, physicians' complaints or problems are brought to the committee for review and appropriate action.

The primary area of concern is that physicians honor their scheduled procedure time and the one-hour OR limit. This requirement does not pose a big problem, because the physicians who use the center regularly realize

Figure 9-2 Crouse-Irving Memorial Hospital Surgery Center Administrative and Organizational Chart

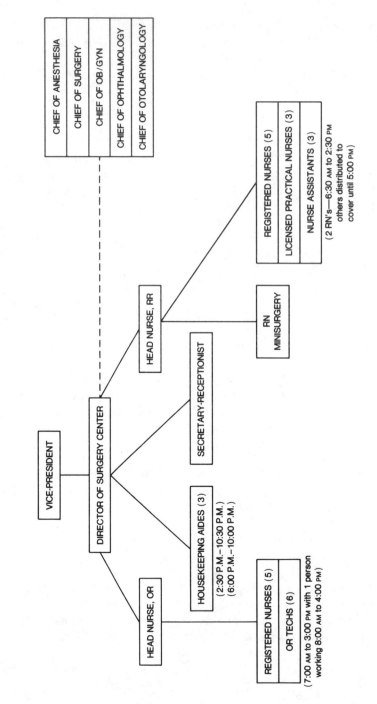

that it is to everyone's advantage (including themselves and their peers) to be on time. The result of these efficiencies and cooperation has financially benefited both patients and the hospital.

CHARGES, PROFITS, AND SAVINGS

When the center opened in 1976, hospital charges were set at $200 and $100 for procedures requiring general and local anesthesia, respectively, and at $60 for laser treatment and minisurgery. These charges covered the use of the facilities; all materials, supplies, and drugs required at the surgery center; and the preoperative CBC and urine tests. Charges for other tests and professional charges were not included.

Cost Containment

The hospital's objective was to provide the surgery center service on a break-even basis. Table 9-3 presents evidence not only that this initial objective was accomplished, but also that the facility produced an increasingly large profit during the first three full years of operation *without increasing patient charges.*

On May 1, 1980, charges were increased to $300 for general anesthesia and $150 for local anesthesia procedures. Laser and minisurgery fees remain at $60. The new charges are obviously not the result of a need to

Table 9-3 Surgery Center Profit and Loss Statement, 1977–81

	1977	*1978*	*1979*	*1980*	*1981*
Income	$851,504	$962,501	$1,001,256	$1,395,313	$1,667,454
Less Surgery Center Allowance	70,346	103,653	3,177	3,514	3,298
Net Income	$781,158	$858,848	$ 998,079	$1,391,799	$1,664,156
Expense					
Salaries	$278,532	$320,020	$ 363,020	$ 417,159	$ 507,519
Fringe Benefits	43,451	48,003	58,265	62,574	76,128
Supplies	78,517	103,012	138,690	214,390	275,790
Rent	270,810	268,793	268,111	274,550	283,656
Indirect Expense	106,267	102,096	114,276	135,614	160,033
Total Expense	$777,577	$841,924	$ 942,362	$1,104,287	$1,303,126
Profit or Loss	$ 3,581	$ 16,924	$ 55,717	$ 287,512	$ 361,030

cover increasing center costs; increased patient volume has taken care of these costs.

The additional profit the surgery center generated in 1980, and is generating now, is used to offset the hospital's increasing inpatient costs. These costs cannot be passed on to the patient or a reimbursement source because of the New York State charge-control law.

The patient and those reimbursement sources that recognize the center have profited also. Hospital charges for surgery center procedures are about only one-fifth of what the charges would be if the same procedure were performed on an inpatient basis. In the first 3¼ years of the surgery center's existence, it is estimated that the savings to patients and third parties exceeded $12 million.

Savings formula

A conservative formula involving existing hospital data and Professional Activities Studies (PAS) data bank input was used to compute this $12 million figure. The PAS data indicated that the fiftieth percentile inpatient length of stay nationally was 2.5 to 3.0 days. The lower figure was multiplied by the hospital's inpatient per diem charge, producing an average inpatient cost per stay. The *maximum* surgery center charge was subtracted from the average inpatient cost per stay to produce an average savings per surgery center patient. This figure was multiplied by the total number of center procedures in order to arrive at what can realistically be considered as a minimum total savings figure.

REIMBURSEMENT EXPERIENCE

Unique Status

Reimbursement has been a twofold problem. First, third party reimbursement sources had some difficulty in recognizing the status of the surgery center itself and the uniqueness of the hospital costs and charges inherent in the operation of the surgery center—the only one of its kind in New York State. Most of these problems are being resolved. Table 9-4 displays the payer mix.

The hospital has adopted a tough posture, insisting on payment by self-pays or reasonable attempts by third parties to arrive at fair reimbursement rates for surgery center procedures. In 1979, for example, one source suddenly began interpreting their surgery center patients' experiences with a technique that benefited the reimburser to an extent the hospital deemed

Table 9-4 Crouse-Irving Memorial Hospital Surgery Center Patient-Reimbursement Mix

Reimbursement Source	Percentage
Blue Cross	41
Commercial Insurance	35
Self-Pay	8
Medicare, Medicaid, No Fault	16

unreasonable. The hospital stopped patients covered by this source from using the surgery center until the problem was resolved.

Staying Power

The second problem has been the greater one, however. It involves Crouse-Irving Memorial Hospital rather than the surgery center, although the success of the center is the cause of the problem.

Early fears that the hospital census or use of the inpatient ORs would decline when the surgery center opened proved groundless. What has occurred, as Table 9-5 shows, is that more patients are staying longer at the hospital. The primary reasons for this are:

- The hospital's surgical facilities are used almost exclusively for major surgery involving more OR time per procedure and a longer length of stay.
- Other beds vacated by short-stay surgery patients are available to patients with critical conditions.

This situation has, in effect, turned much of Crouse-Irving Memorial Hospital into an intensive care facility. This development has placed increased burdens on the hospital staff, particularly the nurses, but the challenge is being met successfully.

The reimbursement challenge generated by the intensive care status has proven more difficult to resolve. Current rates are still being computed by third parties using the same formulas applied to hospitals that do not have surgery centers. Consequently, Crouse-Irving Memorial Hospital has been financially penalized for providing more intensive inpatient care.

The hospital is working with its reimbursement sources, including the state and federal governments, to recognize the situation and adjust compensation accordingly. This situation is not, however, seriously affecting the hospital's financial position. Increased daily patient census and length

Table 9-5 Hospital Statistical Review, 1976–81

	1976	1977	1978	1979	1980	1981
Utilization						
Beds in Service	536	536	536	536	536	536
Average Daily Census	432	456	466	476	494	497
Admissions	24,756	22,815	23,297	24,092	24,898	24,893
Discharges	25,279	23,173	23,358	24,051	24,874	24,892
Percentage of Occupancy	82	85	87	89	92	93
Average Length of Stay (Days)	6.3	7.2	7.3	7.2	7.3	7.3
Services						
Medical-Surgical	8.0	9.3	9.6	9.5	9.4	9.7
Pediatrics	4.2	7.6	7.5	9.0	9.3	9.5
Obstetrics	3.5	3.3	3.6	3.6	3.6	3.5
Nursery	4.0	3.9	3.9	3.8	3.7	3.6
Average Weekend Census	395	427	440	453	459	469
Time per Surgical Procedure	1 hr., 24 min.	1 hr., 42 min.	1 hr., 46 min.	1 hr., 45 min.	1 hr., 44 min.	1 hr., 44 min.

of stay have helped compensate for the difference between appropriate and actual reimbursements. Crouse-Irving Memorial Hospital operated in the black in 1977, 1978, and 1980, and the loss in 1979 was under forty thousand dollars.

FINAL ANSWER

One question frequently raised involves the number of surgery center patients subsequently requiring admission as inpatients. A medical care evaluation committee consisting of nineteen physicians and surgery center staff reviewed all 1979 procedures and found that twenty-seven out of a total of 6,780 patients were admitted to the hospital (see Table 9-6). Seven of the twenty-seven required admission because of bleeding after tonsillectomy and adenoidectomy. Eleven more admissions involved gynecological procedures, and others had postsurgical pain or incomplete recovery from anesthesia.

Only one of the twenty-seven patients was considered in the committee report to have been a poor candidate for ambulatory surgery. Almost all those who had been admitted as inpatients went home the next day.

The advantages outweigh the disadvantages on all fronts. The major question under consideration at this time is whether the hours of the surgery center should be expanded to match increasing demand.

Table 9-6 Surgery Center Visits, 1977–81

	General	Local	Laser	Mini-surgery	Total
1977	4,109	292	330	995	5,726
1978	4,673	346	379	1,113	6,511
1979	4,832	413	385	1,150	6,780
1980	4,999	423	461	1,310	7,193
1981	5,524	315	509	1,149	7,497

	Total OR Hours	Admitted	Average Number of Cases per Day
1977	2,718	36	23
1978	2,771	29	26
1979	2,999	29	27
1980	3,064	32	27
1981	3,317	20	29

The Wichita Minor Surgery Center®: Perspective of the Independent, Freestanding Surgical Center

M. Robert Knapp, M.D., F.A.C.P.

The primary objective in developing a freestanding, independent ambulatory surgical facility should be to meet the community's needs. The hospital in the contemplated area of this surgical facility should regard it as a unit that complements hospital goals and functions for the betterment of the hospital, physicians, community, and, most of all, the patient.

The freestanding, independent ambulatory surgical facility began as the private practitioner's response to the high cost of medical care. Facilities such as the Wichita Minor Surgery Center®, appear to be an appropriate response to the challenge of rendering high-quality surgical care at lower cost to the patient.

REASONS FOR SUCCESS

Because of their small size and limited function, freestanding, independent ambulatory surgical facilities are able to deliver better service at a lower cost than larger health care institutions. By providing specialized facilities for minor surgical procedures, the Minor Surgery Center® and similar facilities are making it possible for hospitals to concentrate on major surgical cases that actually require hospitalization.

From the perspective of cost accounting, there is no justification for patients receiving minor surgical care to pay for the cost of expensive equipment, facilities, or personnel when they do not use them. The patients who use these services should pay for them. By the same token, it is wasteful to expand existing hospital bed space when the need for such additional capacity may well be avoided or reduced by constructing minor surgical facilities at a fraction of the cost.

Adapted from *Journal of Ambulatory Care Management* 1981;3:75–84.

The goal of Minor Surgery Center® and all other freestanding, independent surgical facilities, is to provide physicians and patients with an environment in which the work can be done with a minimum amount of
interference, delay, or distractions. The Minor Surgery Center® is simply
an extension of the physician's office; it has instituted only those regulations that are necessary to record the events that occur in the institution
itself. It seeks to maximize the time during which physicians can concentrate directly on the needs of their patients. A slogan that summarizes the
methodology of the center could be, "Maximizing patient care, minimizing
paper work."

PATIENT TREATMENT

The principal reason for the success of the Minor Surgery Center® is
that the patient is the primary concern. Since the entire organization is
patient oriented, patients encounter only those people who are directly
involved in their care. The orientation is immediately obvious to the
patients the moment they enter the center. Their first encounter with the
nurse is pleasant and reassuring.

Procedures

Laboratory work and directions to patients and their families regarding
procedures are given carefully and quickly. Nurses are encouraged to
study each patient and, if possible, to establish fears and seek to allay
them. All questions are answered courteously and promptly.

The laboratory work at the center is done to determine if the patient is
an adequate anesthetic risk. This work involves a routine urinalysis and
hemoglobin analysis. The patient's temperature, blood pressure, and weight
are recorded. These tests, together with the anesthesiologist's history and
physical examination, provide an adequate basis for determining the physical status of the patient.

The anesthesiologist responsible for administering the anesthetic sees
the patient soon after arrival. The objective is to make this interview brief,
thorough, and above all, reassuring to the patient. The anesthesiologist
examines the patient's heart and lungs and reassures the patient about
care at the center. During this interview and examination the patient may
ask questions, and every effort is made to answer them thoroughly and
completely. The patient is then seen by the surgeon before being taken to
the operating room.

The circulating nurse in charge of the operating room greets the patient
and assures that the patient will be personally taken to the operating room

on the operating room cart. The nurse helps with the transfer to the operating room table and remains in attendance throughout the procedure. All nursing personnel in the operating room are chosen for their outgoing personalities and their skill in surgical nursing. The patient's first encounter with the nurses, therefore, is likely to be warm, friendly, and reassuring. On entering the operating room, the patient is greeted again by the anesthesiologist who offers further reassurance.

Recovery

After surgery, the patient is tranferred to the recovery room. The surgeon's only contact with the patient at the Minor Surgery Center® is during performance of the surgical procedure. The surgeon is not involved with the preoperative examination, admitting procedures, or chart work. The surgeon performs the operation, dictates the procedure while still in the operating room, signs the chart, and writes any specific postoperative orders. Postoperative care, dismissal of the patient, and further chart work are performed by the anesthesiologist.

The anesthesiologist sees the patient again in the recovery room area and dismisses the patient from the Minor Surgery Center® after determining that all is well. The recovery room nurses, too, are chosen because of their competence and proven capacity to be warm, friendly, and reassuring.

The attendance of the anesthesiologist in the recovery room is an important factor in outpatient surgical care. Every effort is made to assure patients that their well-being after leaving the center is of major interest. Each patient is instructed on what to expect while recuperating at home.

If necessary, the anesthesiologist is readily available for consultation with the recovery room nurses. The operating rooms are only a few steps away from the recovery room. If necessary, the patient can be returned to the operating room area for care. As soon as they are receptive, patients are encouraged to take liquid nourishment in the form of soft drinks, coffee, tea, or soup.

The pediatric recovery procedures are somewhat different from those for adults in that the immediate family serves as paramedical personnel. A member of the family is encouraged to be at the child's bedside as soon as vital signs are stable. This means that the child's first encounter postoperatively is with a familiar face, touch, and voice. This presence is not only helpful to the patient but to the parent as well. For liquid nourishment, recuperating children are offered popsicles.

No patient who receives general anesthesia is allowed to leave the Minor Surgery Center® alone. All patients must be accompanied by a friend or relative. The distance from the patient dressing area to the holding area, operating room, recovery room, and exit area are short. Patients seem to appreciate this simplicity of movement. Patients seem to appreciate being able to drive a car within three feet of the front door, park within thirty feet of the building, and be discharged directly into the vehicle within ten feet of the building.

Many patients have had the opportunity to compare service at the Minor Surgery Center® with that of a local hospital. As documented by patient response cards, never have patients reported that the hospital is superior for the ambulatory surgical patient. Obviously, the ability to have an alternative method of surgical care within the community has been met with enthusiasm.

COST CONTRACTS

On August 24, 1972, a contract between Kansas Blue Cross and the Minor Surgery Center® was signed. Kansas Blue Cross covers all services rendered to its subscribers in the Minor Surgery Center®. The charge levied by the Minor Surgery Center® is all-inclusive for each procedure. In this way, Kansas Blue Cross, other insurance carriers, the patient, and the surgeon know in advance exactly what the cost of a given procedure will be. This is guaranteed predictability at its best.

The Health Insurance Association of America (HIAA) was quite encouraging during the genesis of the Minor Surgery Center®. HIAA indicated that the Minor Surgery Center® had complied with the requirements of HIAA's commercial carriers, and recommended coverage of the services in the center's facility to their member companies. Charges to all patients are those facility charges that are negotiated with Kansas Blue Cross.

The Minor Surgery Center® has posted in its lobby the listing of approved surgical procedures (those determined by the Surgical Audit Committee), and after each procedure the facility charge for that service is posted. This list can be characterized as a "menu of surgical facility charges." Physicians fees are *not* a part of this facility charge.

TRANSFER AGREEMENTS

Traditional Beliefs

In the early development of freestanding, independent ambulatory surgical facilities, it was deemed to be appropriate that a facility negotiate transfer agreements with some of its local hospitals. The conventional wisdom of the early 1970s was that there would be frequent transfers of patients from ambulatory surgical facilities to hospitals because of complications arising from surgery. This notion has been shown to be false. It was soon recognized by those involved in freestanding, independent ambulatory surgical care that their facilities could not admit patients to a hospital. The only people who could have admission privileges to a hospital were those on the hospital's medical staff. This restriction, in effect, rendered transfer agreements among these institutions worthless.

No one ever questioned the integrity of those individuals seeking this type of agreement, but it soon became apparent that such agreements simply did not work. Thus came the strategy requiring freestanding, independent ambulatory surgical facilities to permit use of their units only by surgeons and anesthesiologists who had similar privileges in local hospitals. This specification effectively did away with the need for transfer agreements between the surgical facility and the hospital.

Statistical Findings

The nine most frequent surgical procedures done at the Minor Surgery Center® are listed in Table 10-1. Since the Minor Surgery Center® has been in operation, twenty-one thousand patients have been cared for without incident. Of patients coming to the Minor Surgery Center®, 95 percent receive general anesthesia; the remainder are given a local anesthesia. Since the center opened, thirty-one patients have been transferred to hospitals. No transfer was made for emergency reasons.

Every transfer was for pain that was not controllable; suspected perforation of the uterus with admission for observation; or bothersome bleed-

---

Table 10-1 Nine Most frequently Performed Surgical Procedures at the Minor Surgery Center®

Procedure	Number
Myringotomies with Insertion of Drain	3,440
Dental Extractions	3,336
Laparoscopies with Bilateral Tubal Coagulations	2,178
Dilatation and Curettage	2,069
Cystoscopies	1,828
Multiple Lesions	1,290
Vasectomies	633
Breast Mass Excisions	520
Augmentation Mammoplasty	350
Total	15,644

ing that the surgeon believed required continued scrutiny under controlled conditions. Of these thirty-one transfers, only three were made by ambulance; the remainder were made in the automobile of the person accompanying the patient. Thus the incidence of transfers to hospitals reflects the experience of the Freestanding Ambulatory Surgical Association (FASA). The incidence of hospital transfers from the Minor Surgery Center® is one in every 657 patients, or .0015 percent.

The findings of the Minor Surgery Center® as well as of FASA have knocked over the straw man that there would be a 5 percent incidence of transfers to hospitals from units such as the Minor Surgery Center®.[1] Careful selection of patients by the surgeons and the anesthesiologists has ensured the safety of the freestanding, independent ambulatory surgical environment. The data clearly refute the often used argument made by hospitals at Health Systems Agency (HSA) hearings that hospital-sponsored and hospital-based ambulatory surgical facilities have immediate medical support and backup if complications should arise but that this is not the case in the freestanding surgery center. Objective consideration of this statement can only lead to the conclusion that this argument is one based on emotion, not fact.

Professional Staff

The Minor Surgery Center® prides itself on having an all-professional staff. Everyone involved in patient care is either a registered nurse or a physician. Staff includes twenty-two registered nurses. There is also one person who oversees building maintenance and one individual who works in the sterile room for the maintenance and setting up of surgical packs as well as the autoclaving of all supplies. In the office, four full-time persons are employed.

It was discovered by accident that having an all-professional staff in the unit had appeal for other nurses in the Wichita area; high morale engendered by this staffing pattern has brought many applicants seeking jobs for which no vacancies exist. The conditions of employment at the Minor Surgery Center® are so attractive that when an opening for a staff position occurs, the choice can be made from many highly qualified individuals. This broad choice is reassuring to the staff as well as to the employer. Since the Minor Surgery Center® first opened its doors, staff turnover has been minimal.

Orkand Study

In 1972 Congress charged the Department of Health and Human Services (HHS) (then, the Department of Health, Education, and Welfare

[HEW]) (Section 222b, 92–602) with the responsibility of studying and experimenting with the reimbursement of freestanding, independent ambulatory surgical facilities as well as with other ambulatory health care providers. The principal objective was to determine the quality of care rendered in such institutions; the impact on the total health care system of such institutions; and, finally, whether cost savings would accrue to the U.S. taxpayers should freestanding, independent ambulatory surgical facilities and other ambulatory health care providers be reimbursed for their services.

HHS contracted with the Orkand Corporation of Silver Spring, Maryland, to perform the research on freestanding, independent ambulatory surgical facilities. The Orkand study[2] demonstrated that outpatient surgery was significantly less expensive than inpatient surgery; was just as good from a quality standpoint; and, in at least one city, had no adverse impact on hospital occupancy rate. Operations cost less in freestanding, independent units than in freestanding hospital-related units, which in turn were less expensive than conventional hospital inpatient units.

The Orkand study was limited to six freestanding, independent ambulatory surgical facilities in the United States. (The Minor Surgery Center® was one of the units studied.) In all units studied, it was judged that appropriate screening was used for patients; only the low-risk patients were handled via the one-day approach.

In this study, physicians ranked the independent unit highest in terms of their own satisfaction. Patients have shown a similar response. Follow-up studies done by many units affirmed the positive response that patients have to the ambulatory surgical facility that is not affiliated with a hospital.[2] The HHS finally has recognized the worth of the freestanding, independent ambulatory surgical facility as a means of cost containment.

BATTLING TRADITION

The interest of physicians in freestanding, independent ambulatory surgical care has grown over the past ten years. Each success in a given community has led physicians and entrepreneurs in other communities to explore the possibility of constructing such a unit. Many of these physicians consider Washington, D.C., to be the battlefield on which the shape of medical practice will be determined. Too often they fail to recognize that the front lines are in their own backyards. This fact soon becomes apparent, however, when they make their first written application to the local HSA.

Gaining Approval

The application scenario is a familiar one. It has been played and replayed many times in such diverse communities as Las Vegas, Nevada; Buffalo, New York; Fairfax, Virginia; St. Paul, Minnesota; Madison, Wisconsin; Wichita, Kansas; and Phoenix, Arizona. In some instances it has been played out at the comprehensive health planning agencies, which were the predecessors to the HSAs.

In response to the written proposal to the HSA, the local community hospitals immediately counter with ambulatory surgery proposals of their own. For the most part, until application by the independent group, ambulatory surgery in these hospitals will have been relatively uncommon. O'Donovan estimated that "as of 1976, 60 percent of our nation's hospitals have no program of ambulatory surgery."[3]

While the surface issue in the ensuing debate in the HSA centers around the financial pros and cons to the patient and the community, little substantive information is available for the HSA. Matters have improved to the degree that the Orkand Corporation report can be made available as a resource document, but the findings in this report are widely disputed. The gut-level issue that emerges is quite simple: whether to break or continue with tradition.

The furor arises over the existence of any alternative to the present way of doing things. It is a classic case of overkill; hospitals are shooting at a mosquito with a cannon. The real problem could be anxiety over larger and more threatening changes that inevitably lie ahead. There must be a willingness to experiment if solutions to major health care questions are to be found; and these solutions cannot be at the expense of private citizens.

Seton's Struggle

A classic example of the struggle can be found in Buffalo, New York. Two surgeons, Lewis Cloutier and John R. F. Ingall, proposed to the HSA of Western New York the construction of a freestanding, independent ambulatory surgical facility—the Seton Ambulatory Surgical Center. The application for the Seton project was submitted to the State Health Department in 1976 and was subsequently approved by the HSA of Western New York. Cloutier and Ingall went through the labyrinthine process of attempting to demonstrate conclusively to the HSA that there was a need for such a surgical facility in Erie County.

After the doctors' successful battle on the local level, the HSA of Western New York forwarded its recommendation of approval of the

Seton Center to the State Hospital Review and Planning Council and the State Public Health Council. Both councils act as advisory groups to the State Health Commission. The two councils ruled that there was not a need for such an ambulatory center in Erie County.

Marianne K. Adams, Executive Secretary of the Public Health Council, explained: "The health care delivery system in New York and western New York is over expanded, particularly in terms of excess hospital beds. While the Seton project would add no new beds to the system, it would expand and over expand the system further" (*Buffalo Evening News*, Feb. 12, 1978). One must wonder how, in the face of the Orkand study, such a conclusion could possibly have ben reached.

The Seton predicament has a Catch-22 ring to it: The project could help cut back on an overexpanded system, but because the system is already overexpanded, it will not be approved. The Seton Ambulatory Surgical Center is not yet in existence, and it is not clear whether the battle will continue.

Those health care professionals interested in freestanding, independent ambulatory surgical facilities and their continued development throughout the country must not let the Orkand report die in the HHS. A comment carried in a recent article outlined the fate of such reports—"large, voluminous and forgotten."[4(p.687)] Those same professionals will continue to assert that freestanding, independent ambulatory surgical care costs less, achieves the same high quality of surgical care achievable in the hospital setting, and has no measurable impact on the hospitals within a community. Perhaps the greatest service that such facilities perform for a community is to prevent construction of further hospital bed space.

ACCREDITATION

Until early 1979 the Society for the Advancement of Free-Standing Ambulatory Surgical Care had conducted an accreditation program for the freestanding, independent ambulatory surgical facilities. This program had been ongoing since 1975. Twenty-seven surgical facilities had met the standards of the society and had been accredited. With the passage of time and the growing recognition of the importance of ambulatory heatlh care as a cost-containment device, a need for a broader accreditation mechanism was perceived.

Concern for high standards in the delivery of ambulatory health care has led to the formation of the Accreditation Association for Ambulatory Health Care (AAAHC). The sponsoring organizations of this pioneer group are the American College Health Association; the American Group Practice Association; the Group Health Association of America, Inc.; Medical Group Management Association; the National Association of Community Health Centers; and the Freestanding Ambulatory Surgical Association. This new association began the accreditation of ambulatory health care facilities on May 1, 1979.

Quoting from the bylaws of the AAAHC, the purpose of the association is: A. To establish standards for the operation of ambulatory health care facilities and services; B. To conduct surveys and accreditation programs that will promote and identify high quality, cost effective ambulatory health care programs and services; C. to recognize compliance with standards by issuance of certificates of accreditation.

Those involved in ambulatory surgical care have chosen to cast their lot with some other providers in the ambulatory health care field. They have done this because of an unshakeable belief in the validity of what they are doing. The quality of ambulatory surgical care is upgraded through such an accreditation mechanism. Such action bodes well for the future of this newly developing area of surgical care, as well as for all others within the orbit of ambulatory health care. By the end of AAAHC's second fiscal year (April 30, 1981), about twenty-five ambulatory surgical centers will have been surveyed. At present, fourteen freestanding, independent ambulatory surgical facilities have received accreditation from the AAAHC.

FINAL ANALYSIS

The greatest problem facing advocates of the freestanding, independent ambulatory surgical concept is the problem of obstructionism. They believe, without any doubt, that they have more than proven their point. They have shown that high-quality surgical care can be delivered for less money within the freestanding, independent ambulatory surgical environment. Yet the drama of obstructionism has been performed throughout the United States in virtually every community in which a freestanding, independent ambulatory surgical facility is functioning and in many communities in which attempts to establish such facilities have been successful.

Ambulatory surgical care is not a new new concept. It is one that has once again found its proper place as an acceptable option in patient care. Those who operate freestanding, independent surgical units are convinced that their units take better care of patients, patients' families, and attending physicians than do the large, impersonal hospitals. They believe that small is better.

Freestanding, independent ambulatory surgical units are single-purpose institutions whose job it is to operate smoothly, efficiently, and with little fuss. They have demonstrated their capacities to save the time of both the physician and the patient. They also save the patient money without compromising the quality of surgical care. The future for freestanding, independent ambulatory surgical units is a bright one, and the properly planned and built facility will demonstrate that it is an asset to its community and to the entire health care system of that community.

REFERENCES

1. Bruns K:; Annual data report. Read before the Freestanding Ambulatory Surgery Association Meeting, Las Vegas, February 1980.
2. *Comparative Evaluation of Cost, Quality and System Effect of Ambulatory Surgery Performed in Alternative Settings.* US Dept. of Health, Education, and Welfare publication No. TR–772–102. Health Care Financing Administration, Office of Policy Planning and Research, December 1977.
3. O'Donovan TR: *Ambulatory Surgical Centers, Development and Management.* Germantown, Md, Aspen Systems Corp. 1976, p XIV.
4. Greenberg DS: Reportitis: Not so trival a disorder. *N Engl J Med* 1979; 300:687–688.

Chapter 11

Ambulatory Surgery from a Patient's Perspective

Eleanor Nealon

The trend to ambulatory surgery is spreading rather complacently across the United States. Meanwhile, it should not be forgotten—even with the diminutive sound of this "short-stay" surgery—that a terrified, ill-prepared patient is a poor surgical risk, and that an unhappy, angry patient is a poor consumer advocate.

Although the trend may have the enthusiastic backing of health professions, administrators, and third party payers, the consumer is a central part of the equation. Patients' perspectives and experiences count. From humane, ethical, and economic viewpoints, it is important to recognize patients' concerns and to meet their needs.

Essential ingredients go into the successful packaging of ambulatory surgery as a positive experience for man, woman, or child. These ingredients range from proper preparation and reassurance to quality medical care and postoperative follow-up. Compressing a surgical experience into a short period of time with early release from the hospital does not eliminate the necessity for sensitivity and supportive care, comfortable facilities, and adequate information. As with any health care delivery, the important question to keep in mind is: What is this experience like from the *patient's perspective?* The two examples that follow will illustrate this point.

TWO EXAMPLES OF AMBULATORY PATIENT TREATMENT

Elise Kawalski (the real names of patients have been changed) was thirty-five and wanted to have children. When her physician recommended dilatation and curettage (D & C) to rule out malignancy as the cause of medical symptoms she was having, she was not only afraid that she had cancer, but also that this procedure would lead to a hysterectomy. He

165

explained the D & C could be done as an ambulatory procedure; she could return home afterward if all went as expected.

Elise dutifully went to the hospital several days before surgery for blood tests, x-ray, urinalysis, and EKG. Although the visit required her to take time off from work, she understood the necessity for these tests. On the morning of surgery, she got up, dressed, and left for the hospital at 6:30 A.M. while it was still dark. Having followed the instructions not to drink any liquids or wear any cosmetics, she felt tired with no coffee, her mouth was dry with no water, and she felt naked and ugly with no makeup.

The admissions office took her to the surgery rooms of the obstetrics and gynecology department. Surprised to find herself in the labor and delivery room area, she was told that D & Cs and Cesarean sections were performed in the same area.

She changed her clothes and nervously waited in a room with two beds. Several people, including the anesthesiologist, came in to check her. After more than an hour, a nurse escorted her to one of the surgery rooms. She shuffled along in her paper slippers and oversized gown. She gritted her teeth, walked in, and got up on the table. The lights were bright, and she could look around the room at the green-gowned, masked figures. She lay down on the hard metal table and could feel herself shaking from a chill. A nurse put a blanket over her.

The surgeon came in and chatted briefly with her. Then the anesthesiologist took her arm, and soon she began to slip into unconsciousness. She awoke in the recovery room groggy and in pain. Her surgeon said that she was doing fine and that the results of her pathology tests would be ready later. Then he was gone. She was moved to a darkened room, where another woman had also just returned from surgery.

Elise welcomed sleep, but awoke from pain and the sound of a woman in the next room screaming in labor. The patient beside her was upset because she had been ringing for a nurse but no one had come. The nurses were busy helping with the delivery of several babies. Before Elise was discharged, she had to lie in the darkness with her fear of a hysterectomy, which was heightened by the constant reminder of other women around her giving birth. Her fear was made nightmarish by the screams of the woman in labor that floated through her semiconsciousness as she alternately slept and awoke.

In contrast, Mrs. Sylvia Lipson's ambulatory surgery for a breast biopsy was handled with sensitivity. When her internist told her she had a breast lesion, she was shocked. She was referred to a surgeon and told not be too alarmed, that it probably was not malignant. "I thought they were just telling me that," she said. On the other hand, she couldn't believe it was happening to her.

Although the surgeon was informative and gentle, Mrs. Lipson was frightened. She and her husband decided to go ahead with the biopsy.

When Sylvia went to the hospital on the day of the surgery, she found that she had been given a private room complete with a television and bathroom. She changed her clothes for surgery in comfort. The surgery, scheduled for 9:30 A.M., was rescheduled for 10:40 A.M. It was hard to wait, but the fact that her husband and a friend were allowed to wait with her helped. The nurses were thoughtful; they seemed to understand her terror.

When the time came for her to go in a wheelchair to the operating room, the short trip seemed like miles. What about the operating room itself? "That was scary; it's awful," she laughed. Mrs. Lipson's surgeon met her there, and a resident asked some questions she had already answered. The presence of the resident caused a momentary upset. Sylvia was anxious to complete the biopsy, and now she had a new fear. "Are you turning me over to this young doctor?" she asked her surgeon with concern. She was assured that her concern was unfounded. Although these questions were repetitious, they are routine in a teaching hospital.

Her surgeon explained that she would receive a local anesthetic by injection and that she would experience no discomfort. "I'll tell you everything as I go along," he reassured. A screen was placed in front of her face so that she could not see the procedure. Earlier her surgeon had asked her if she liked opera. "Of course," she had answered. At this point, the operating room staff started a music tape of Pavarotti that played softly.

"I love music," she smiled, remembering the thoughtful touch. "It certainly relaxed and distracted me. It was wonderful. I couldn't get over it."

The surgeon thought he had found a benign cyst. He informed Sylvia that he would have the pathology report in a few days. "I knew nothing more would happen to me that day," she said. Her surgeon prescribed a pain medication and she and her husband went to lunch before she returned home to put on ice packs.

"Everything was geared to make me comfortable," she recalled about the ambulatory surgery unit. "They treated me the same as if I were having major surgery."

The two preceding patient experiences highlight differences in sensitivity to patient needs within the same institution in units run by different departments. Both patients were treated in an ambulatory setting, and both approached their procedures with some trepidation. In the first case, the patient's psychological fears, as well as physical discomfort, were all but ignored. The second situation, however, provides a practical example in meeting a patient's mental and physical requirements in an ambulatory setting by combining the requisite skills with sensitivity to and awareness of the patient's needs.

AMBULATORY SURGERY FOR ADULTS

Patients generally seem receptive to the idea of ambulatory surgery. A major question patients ask is, Docs my insurance cover the procedure? Patients should determine this. They should also understand that a short-stay hospitalization is economical because it avoids not only inpatient room costs but also miscellaneous charges that add up such as television rental. Patients find that they are pleased with the lower expense of short-stay hospitalization as opposed to an inpatient admission; and that with proper preparation and instruction, it is likely they will be more comfortable at home. Although most people are happy to avoid staying in the hospital, there are areas of anxiety and concern for some that need to be discussed.

It is common sense that short-stay hospitalization does not negate the pain, discomfort, or fear normally associated with a particular surgical procedure (e.g., a breast biopsy). The private physician should inform patients about what to expect and instruct them in how to deal with events associated with the procedure.

Patients often expect an experience to be far worse than it is. They should have the opportunity to discuss any fears of surgery itself or anesthesia (general or local). They also need to understand that medically they are good candidates for ambulatory surgery. It may help to explain to some patients who are uneasy that surgical care in ambulatory units is not compromised. As Frank C. Buxton, executive officer of the operating rooms at Georgetown University Hospital, said, "In a short-stay unit, the purpose is to do all the things that you should do for a patient. It offers the same quality of care in a more expedient manner."

Certain patients may fear losing the security blanket of longer-term postoperative professional observation, or perhaps unconsciously may resent being robbed of the "adventure" of staying overnight in a hospital, with the accompanying sympathy of friends and relatives. All patients need reassurance that they will be discharged only if they meet the necessry medical criteria and can manage their own care. The regulation that a responsible adult must take the patient home is relatively easy to accept for those patients with families, but it may pose problems for others. Even with family support, it is important to alert patients to plan ahead and avoid the situation of Mrs. Brown, who complained, "It's very inconvenient for me to go home today, Doctor. My husband is away. Oh, couldn't I please stay?''

On the other hand, patients should be aware that in some cases, though rarely, they may have to remain in the hospital overnight. When scheduling ambulatory procedures, there is usually time to plan for contingencies. The system should also maintain a reasonable degree of flexibility to allow for admitting certain hardship cases in which a patient lacks immediate postoperative care or an adequate home situation.

Undoubtedly there are some inconveniences involved. General anesthesia patients usually must take time from work or activities to come in advance for blood work and other tests. Although such tests may necessitate another trip to the hospital, this minor inconvenience is less stressful than waiting until the day of surgery and discovering at the last minute that surgery has to be postponed because of a test result.

Ambulatory surgery is probably most difficult for single individuals living alone, who may hesitate to impose on friends to bring them home, manage with groceries, and so on. These patients may believe that the hospital has transferred its responsibility unfairly to them, causing them to be dependent on others. Patients also experience tension, real or imagined, about the closing time of the unit. Is it before the end of the workday, making it necessary for someone to leave work early to meet them? With proper preparation and thought, difficulties can be worked out, possibly ahead of time.

Frank C. Buxton stressed that a patient's surgical experience begins with the physician and the physician's office staff. They are the ones who set the stage and explain why a procedure can be done on an ambulatory basis. They put the case in perspective and give the necessary patient instructions. A comprehensive list of written instructions for general anesthesia patients prepared either by the physician or the hospital is easiest to remember. If they are not inpatients, patients may decide that they do not have to abide by hospital rules as closely. A cavalier attitude also may develop about arriving on time at the hospital because patients may not understand how their tardiness could delay the operating room schedule. Again, preparation and education can prevent these problems.

Preparation continues in the hospital on the day of surgery. An alert and supportive staff can recognize apprehension and try to lower a patient's anxiety. Questions should be encouraged. Claire T. West, R.N., director of nursing, department of operating rooms, at Georgetown University Hospital, pointed out that some patients are intimidated by surgery and some do not want too much information. However, every patient should be encouraged to ask questions. From the consumer point of view they're entitled to the best service. She added that complaints tend to be mostly time oriented.

Waiting is probably the most difficult time for patients, especially when surgery schedules run late. It is important that patients wait in comfortable surroundings with an atmosphere of individualized care. They do not like to wander around in gowns in front of strangers and with no room or place for their belongings.

The best situation, if possible, is a private room with bath facilities and a television where family or friends can join the patient if desired. (Parents should be required to stay with children.) The worst situation is an environment with little privacy and a sense of being "one of the herd." As well as being uncomfortable, this atmosphere may create doubts as to the quality of the medical care. It is alarming for a patient waiting for surgery to perceive the unit as a makeshift or ancillary facility.

Basically, patients need a proper place to change clothes, respect for privacy, access to clean bathroom facilities, and a secure feeling that the staff is approachable. It is helpful if the staff is aware that seemingly small incidents can terrify an already anxious patient.

For example, Alice Hogan, thirty-five, was scheduled for surgery with a general anesthetic. She had only been in the hospital emergency department as a child and never had surgery or anesthesia. "I was scared to death," she said. "I had never been unconscious." Because her physician had not told her anything about what to expect, she called the clinic and said she was coming in and was anxious about it; could they tell her step-by-step what would happen. She was grateful when they did.

The morning of surgery, as she waited in her green gown with her clothes stowed in a locker, a nurse took a blood test from her arm and walked away. A few minutes later Alice looked down and panicked at the sight of blood dripping down her arm. She ran after the nurse, crying, "Here, look, look!" The incident heightened her fear of the impending surgery.

To make matters worse for Alice, in the operating room when the needle for anesthesia was inserted in her arm, she felt a tingling. "Stop it," she said, "there's something wrong." The anesthesiologist adjusted the needle and told her to count backwards from 100. She struggled with the worry that when she was unconscious, she could not tell anyone if something went wrong.

Looking at the types of procedures now handled in ambulatory surgery programs, probably the most difficult one that a patient faces psychologically is a breast biopsy (either with local or general anesthetic). Paul J. Melluzzo, M.D., assistant professor of surgery, Georgetown University Hospital, pointed out that ambulatory surgery for breast biopsy does not remove the natural fears and questions regarding the procedure. Women have the same apprehensions about their diagnosis and prognosis, whether or not they are admitted to the hospital as inpatients. If they do not require hospitalization before or after the biopsy, however, he thinks that fact may somewhat reduce the anixety. Often, the knowledge that the physician will not go ahead with a mastectomy that day also alleviates some of the tension.

The nursing staff in the Georgetown Hospital's ambulatory unit tries to give particular support to breast biopsy patients. Lori Hess, R.N., assistant nursing coordinator there, thinks that at such times "husbands don't know what to do. It's a great strain. A wife is brave in front of a husband but when he leaves, the nurses are still there and she can voice her feelings to them." Of course, some women will be discharged from the unit knowing that they probably have cancer, and others will still be uncertain as they wait for pathology results.

Many patients, whatever the procedure, understandably have fears and questions about anesthesia. Before surgery with a general anesthetic, patients should have the opportunity to ask the anesthesiologist questions (before meeting in the operating room), and be reassured about the anesthesia as much as possible. Giving preoperative medication varies by hospital unit and patient case. The support of the nursing staff and the physicians could probably provide as much reassurance to many patients as could presedation—and with longer "time-released action."

When a patient faces local anesthesia, the fear of slipping into unconsciousness vanishes but other worries can arise. A bad experience in a dentist's office or an emergency department can be dredged up. Two fears may be: (1) I will be awake and know what's going on. Will that be terrible? and, (2) What if the shot doesn't work and I can feel the surgery? Local anesthetics, therefore, also call for explanation. There are now aids, such as taped music, to distract the patient. Many patients say afterward, "the surgery wasn't as bad as I thought."

During surgery with a local anesthetic, Dr. Melluzzo said, surgeons try to anticipate which patient may hyperventilate or faint. They talk to the patient during the procedure and explain what's happening. "You may feel some sensation now—a sting," they may say as the anesthesia is injected. "Let us know if you feel anything else and we can inject more." This approach gives the patient joint control with the surgeon. It is a cooperative effort.

Patients who are "local standbys" may be reassured knowing that if a local is not sufficient, they will receive a general anesthesia; or they may feel uneasy about the uncertainty and expect the local not to work.

For some patients, having a cyst removed in ambulatory surgery provides them with an interesting look at the operating room, and they go through surgery with little discomfort. For others, however, who face more anxiety-producing procedures, the waiting period and the trip to the operating room are frightening. The operating room is an awesome and somewhat hostile place for ''xenophobes'' (which most of the public would be in that setting). What reassures them is a sense of the expertise that lies behind the array of impersonal technology. Above all, patients want quality medical care without complications, whether it is for a hernia, rectal polyps, or a face lift. They should never be given the impression that an ambulatory surgical facility is like a carry-out place or a second-rate assembly line.

It may be wiser, in fact, to publicize or make readily available a list of ambulatory surgery programs (hospital-sponsored and independent) that have been legitimately approved or accredited. Probably few people— health professions or the general public—are aware that a list of approved centers may be obtained, for example from the Joint Commission on Accreditation of Hospitals or the Accreditation Assocation for Ambulatory Health Care, Inc.

Quality care, of course, extends postoperatively. Laurence Chaparell was brought from the recovery room to a private room where he rested, letting the anesthesia wear off. It was comfortable and the staff gave him good care. His surgery to remove a large growth on the back of his neck had lasted longer than expected—two hours. When he awoke, he was dizzy but thought that was normal. Later in the afternoon, after being checked medically, his physician discharged him with pain medication and a telephone number to call if there was any problem. Mr. Chaparell was instructed about the drain in his neck and told it would be removed the next day. He was happy to go home. ''You feel more comfortable with relatives around you,'' he said. He left the unit with confidence. ''I had the feeling that the staff cared, that everything would be in order.''

The continuum of instructing patients before, during, and after surgery is important. If admission is required, an explanation is needed to put the situation in perspective so as not to unduly alarm the patient. Such treatment would benefit one young girl who recently had heart arrythmias during surgery, was subsequently admitted for observation, but was relased the next day.

A number of patients are concerned that they will not be able to manage going home or will be released too early. Here the physician and staff can reinforce the fact that they are all right to go home and that they do meet discharge criteria. In some ambulatory units, patients are aggravated by the pressure to leave the unit quickly. In certain cases this pressure may be a misconception on the part of the patient, but not in all instances. One patient who had general anesthesia in an otherwise excellent unit—which stayed open, she later found out, until 6:30 P.M.—was told by a staff member that she should be out of the unit by 4:00 P.M. She had some pain and grogginess, and was upset because arrangements had been made to pick her up at 5:30 P.M. It was disturbing to have to call a friend and ask him to leave work early to pick her up. This situation created needless tension for all concerned.

Another patient, Louise Semmes, received preoperative medication (morphine and seconal, as she recalled) before plastic surgery on her face. The last thing she remembered was being put on the operating table for a local anesthetic. She awoke to hear a nurse saying, "You didn't have the procedure. You can wake up now." A resident with poor English told her she was not able to have the surgery because she had an adverse drug reaction. She felt pressured to leave the unit and had the impression that the nurses' attitude was, "You didn't have the procedure, so go home."

Louise had planned to leave at 6:00 P.M. but ended up waiting in the emergency department waiting room at 4:00 P.M. She went home feeling "spacey" and depressed. A "total drug down," she called it. She left right before her physician returned to see her.

Some patients are released to families or friends who are mystified or apprehensive about taking them home. The physician and medical staff can smooth the exit. If major responsibility for postoperative care is transferred to the patient and the patient's relatives and friends, there is a concomitant need for instruction and reassurance before discharge from the ambulatory unit. It is the main role of the personal physician to instruct about care; to schedule necessary follow up; and, along with any prescription for pain, say, "Call if you need me."

AMBULATORY CARE FOR CHILDREN

When children have ambulatory surgery, both patients and their parents need to be considered. Mary E. Robinson, M.D., director of the department of child life at Children's Hospital National Medical Center, said that it is better to prepare children psychologically in advance for a surgical experience so that they can digest the information and ask quetions. Preparation of family and patient is inadequate if done too close to the time of surgery. The risk is that a child has already developed too many fears.

Robinson said that a hospital is responsible for: (1) preadmission orientation, (2) orientation at the time of surgery, and (3) having a staff that is responsive to the patient's fears.

Children's Hospital National Medical Center offers orientation tours prior to surgery. There are printed materials and a puppet show about the hospital, which is a strange and scary world for youngsters. (Children do not understand operating rooms. It is helpful to explain the situation on their own level of understanding in accordance with their age and personality.)

For the ambulatory surgery unit, which only takes general anesthesia cases at Children's Hospital, patients have blood work done in advance, then arrive the day of surgery at the admissions office. Here they are examined and change their clothes. Then children meet the anesthesiologist in the waiting room, which is a playroom. Most patients do not receive preoperative sedation. "Rather than presedate, we give them their parents," Robinson said. Whether or not children are presedated, where they wait and with whom is important in order to ease anxiety. As Robinson pointed out, children on a stretcher in a crowded corridor may hear "appalling" things and think they refer to them even if they do not.

Children are afraid of needles and pain and may not like being put to sleep. At Children's Hospital, parents accompany their children to an induction room, where anesthesia is started, and stay until the child goes to sleep. Parents remain at the hospital for the day. After surgery, children are moved to the main recovery room and then to an ambulatory recovery unit from which they are discharged. It is difficult for some parents to see their children return from surgery still groggy, with an intravenous needle still intact, and perhaps vomiting bloody mucus. "It's a stressful time, but we feel kids do better with the parents," Robinson said.

Parents may also fear their child will be abruptly discharged at a certain unit closing time, and they need reassurance that there are specific discharge criteria. They may worry about the medical apsects of caring for their children at home. (Alert staff members can call the physician's attention to a parent who seems unable to handle the situation.) At Children's Hospital, parents receive a discharge sheet and physician's instructions. "It's a lot of responsibility to parents," Robinson granted. "Most want it—they want to do as much as they can for their child . . . and they should not feel alone in it."

Robinson pointed out the amazing rapidity with which most children recover from anesthesia and are ready to leave the hospital. She suggested, however, that whoever brings the child home may want to have another adult along. On the way home, the child may vomit and need assistance, or may simply need to snuggle up to the parent.

Looking at ways to improve ambulatory surgery for children, Robinson made the following comments:

- It is essential for the referring physician or surgeon to assume preparation of the patient and not leave the emotional preparation to the hospital, because there is no time.

- It is important for the anesthesiologist to make a brief contact with the child in a "neutral" area like a playroom, and not wait until the meeting in the operating room.
- Hospitals should have a person (a nurse or patient educator) in the admitting area to answer patient questions or assist the patient who is unduly upset. This staff person could take notice of a particularly anxious child and call an anesthesiologist or other physician to come and talk to that patient. (At Children's Hospital, if the situation is serious enough, the operating schedule will be rearranged.)

And how do some consumers look at ambulatory surgery for their children? One mother brought her son home after a hernia repair. "Kids probably do better at home," she acknowledged, "but it was terrible. He was sick and had pain. I was up all night and scared he would rip his stitches. I talked to the doctor about ten times."

Another mother, Genevieve Talbot, said her sons have had several ambulatory surgeries. She felt this approach lowered the trauma and was easier emotionally on the child, but "a little scary for the mother." It was frightening for her to see her child go limp with anesthesia, although she believed it was important to stay with him. After each operation, the physician gave her instructions and she asked numerous questions.

"It's incumbent on the doctor to give instructions, but you're still scared," she said. The last time she brought her son home after eye surgery, his eye oozed blood and he got sick in the car. But Tommy felt better when he reached their front door. "Like any of us," she said, "he was glad to be home."

Surgery—even ambulatory surgery—can be difficult for children or adults. There are ways to make the experience easier and better for those concerned, but this requires mentally stepping into the patient's place and looking at the surgery from that perspective in order to get an essential understanding of the person's needs and how these can best be filled. Claire West, R.N., at Georgetown Hospital, said that the most welcome comment health professionals can hear from a patient is, "You treated me like a real person, not like an operation."

Chapter 12

Ambulatory Surgery and Health Insurance

Steven Sieverts

It is axiomatic that health insurance plans that provide coverage for surgery performed during hospitalizations should also provide coverage for equivalent surgery performed on an outpatient basis. Ambulatory surgery can be both safer and less costly than inpatient surgery, and it should be supported. To deny coverage for properly defined ambulatory surgery is to push patients unnecessarily into hospitalization, because medical care does respond to financial factors.

This chapter discusses this subject from the standpoint of Blue Cross and Blue Shield, the nonprofit health service plans across the United States that provide health insurance through arrangements that include contracts among the plans; the institutional providers of services; and, to the extent achievable, the practicing physicians. Although references will be made to policies and practices recommended by the Blue Cross/Blue Shield Association (the national association of the Blue Cross/Blue Shield plans), the specific focus will be on Blue Cross/Blue Shield of Greater New York and its extensive experience with ambulatory surgery.

Blue Cross/Blue Shield of Greater New York serves over 8 million non-Medicare subscribers who live in the seventeen downstate counties of New York, or who live in northern New Jersey and western Connecticut and are covered through New York-based employment. About half of that total is covered by the plan for physician services as well as hospital services, and a growing number is also protected by Blue Cross/Blue Shield's major medical policies.

The plan's medical-surgical benefits have always covered surgical procedures regardless of where they were performed. The advent of organized ambulatory surgery programs at hospitals and freestanding, independent facilities was therefore easily accommodated by the Blue Shield (physician-service benefit) programs of the plan. The fees paid for surgeons' services and the benefit definitions are the same whether the procedure is done in-hospital, in an ambulatory surgical facility of a hospital, in a freestanding, independent unit, in a surgeon's office, or elsewhere.

"Outpatient surgery" institutional-service benefits were explicitly added to the plan's hospitalization (or Blue Cross) contracts in 1970, covering a generally defined range of surgical procedures in hospital outpatient departments. This addition was intended as a basic liberalization of Blue Cross/Blue Shield's hospital emergency room benefits, expanding them to include the institutional aspects of minor nonemergency procedures performed in outpatient departments and clinics. Such procedures ranged from the removal of sutures or casts and the excision of minor cysts or warts, to relatively more extensive procedures, such as diagnostic dilatation and curettage and various minor orthopedic procedures. The benefit was subsequently reinterpreted also to cover outpatient transfusions and certain major invasive diagnostic procedures, such as thoracentesis and amniocentesis.

GUIDELINES

In 1977—based in part on a positive experience in providing coverage experimentally at the New York City facilities of Planned Parenthood—the plan's board of directors adopted a set of guidelines[1] for freestanding, independent ambulatory care facilities that wanted to have contracts with Blue Cross/Blue Shield of Greater New York. Generally following the prototype guidelines recommended by the Blue Cross Association,[2] this promulgation established standards of quality, safety, and cost for such services. The services covered by the plan conformed to the same definitions used to define outpatient surgery at hospitals.

In 1981 these guidelines were revised and made more specific for freestanding, independent ambulatory surgical facilities, as differentiated from other ambulatory care units that were not primarily surgical in nature, such as freestanding, independent birthing centers. The current guidelines[3] of Blue Cross/Blue Shield of Greater New York are as follows:*

> 1) The facility should be appropriately licensed, should meet the standards of the relevant accrediting body (if any), and should be approved for operation under the appropriate legislation of the state in which the facility is located.
>
> 2) The facility should have a written agreement with one or more nearby general hospitals, covering such matters as the transfer of patients requiring inpatient care, procedures for quality assurance, and the responsibility of the principal back-up hospital or

---

*Reprinted with the permission of Blue Cross and Blue Shield of Greater New York.

some other appropriate entity to exercise surveillance of those procedures.

3) The facility should operate efficiently, should provide patient care which is appropriate, and meets accepted medical standards, and should seek consistently to deliver service of high quality. There should be appropriate permanent facilities, equipment, scheduling, nursing staff, and support staff for the health services it provides.

4) The facility should be governed by a clearly identified governing authority with full legal responsibility for the conduct of the institution and the services rendered. There should be a chief executive officer with delineated responsibility for the management of the institution in accordance with policies established by the governing authority.

5) The facility should have a formally organized medical staff functioning under rules and regulations established by the governing authority, including procedures for delineating the scope of professional practice permitted for each member of the medical staff by specific action of the governing authority. The members of the medical staff should each have appointments with equivalent delineated privileges at one or more hospitals in the area; a majority should have active medical staff appointments at the principal back-up hospital, if feasible.

6) The governing body, through its medical staff and chief executive officer, should be responsible for the conduct of periodic and ongoing utilization review and medical care evaluation in a manner equivalent to that required of an accredited hospital.

7) The facility should be housed in quarters that conform to all appropriate safety and fire laws in force in the jurisdiction in which it operates. The facility should be maintained and designed to protect the patients.

8) The facility should maintain current and complete medical records for each patient. Such records should be available for reference. If the patient must be admitted to an inpatient facility because of complications, a complete copy of the medical record should be sent immediately to the admitting hospital.

9) No operative procedure should be performed before the appropriate history, physical, and diagnostic examinations have been performed. The results of such examinations should be entered in the patient's medical record prior to surgery.

10) The facility should have immediately available the necessary equipment and personnel trained to deal with emergencies that might arise in the course of the facility's programs. When medically indicated, at least one physician should be present when patients are being treated at the facility. No patient should be discharged without a physician's approval. At discharge, arrangements should be made to ensure follow-up care for the patient, if such is medically appropriate.

11) The facility should not maintain inpatient beds for overnight stays, should not routinely offer emergency medical care, and should not attempt to provide services which exceed its certified purposes or which it is not able to deliver safely with high quality.

The introductory chapter of this book describes the standards of the Joint Commission on Accreditation of Hospitals (JCAH) with respect to ambulatory surgical units.[4] For facilities not accredited by the JCAH, the plan itself applies those standards in evaluating the facility for possible contracting status. In all cases site visits by the plan's health care programs and medical departments are made prior to board actions approving the execution of contracts with these facilities; equivalent standards and approval procedures are followed by the plan when hospitals, alcoholism rehabilitation centers, and other facilities seek contractual participating status with the plan.

REIMBURSEMENT

For hospital-based routine outpatient surgery services, the plan's reimbursement rates are the same as those established for the emergency departments of the hospital. That is, under the prospective reimbursement methodology of Blue Cross/Blue Shield of Greater New York, as approved each year by the state's Departments of Health and Insurance, audited average costs per emergency room visit are determined for each "base year"; rates per visit are calculated for the "rate year" by multiplying that average cost by a two-year trend factor reflecting inflation in the economy. Because the quantity of emergency room visits to area hospitals by the public is generally increasing—thus tending to lower the inflation-adjusted cost per visit—the prospectively determined rates are usually at or above the actual costs incurred by the hospital in providing these services.

In the late 1970s, it gradually became apparent that ambulatory surgery in hospital outpatient departments was progressing beyond relatively uncomplicated excisions, cast removals, and transfusions to more complex procedures of many kinds. This trend reflected the development of less traumatic anesthesia media, and the growing realization that early ambulation and return to the home could produce quicker recoveries, fewer postoperative complications, and significant savings in costs.

The plan's practice of lumping together the total number of outpatient surgery procedures with hospital emergency room services thus was becoming anomalous. Although the services provided to the average emergency room patient are not quantitatively very different from the services provided to a patient in a similar facility undergoing a minor surgical procedure, this situation may not be the case when more extensive procedures are performed. This difference became particularly apparent when hospitals began developing special programs, facilities, and staff for ambulatory surgery involving general anesthesia and postoperative recovery, as well as a greater surgical capacity.

The plan subsequently developed the option for hospitals to apply for special reimbursement rates for ambulatory surgery. These rates are calculated on the same basis as emergency room visits rate: base year costs per surgical procedure are trended forward to establish current rates. A ceiling of double the hospital's prospectively determined inpatient per diem rate is imposed on the ambulatory surgery rate. As of the beginning of 1982, about one-third of the plan's participating hospitals had established ambulatory surgery reimbursement rates. Only a few low-volume programs in their beginning phase had rates affected by the ceiling; typically, and not surprisingly, the ambulatory surgery rate for a hospital is similar to its per diem rate.

Blue Cross/Blue Shield of Greater New York's outpatient surgery benefit under its hospitalization contracts now covered: surgical procedures in which the special resources of a hospital (or freestanding) ambulatory surgery program were appropriate; and the more minor kinds of outpatient procedures that are ordinarily done in less specialized settings, such as hospital clinics, emergency department treatment rooms, and physicians' private offices. There was thus a need to differentiate between outpatient surgery not requiring an ambulatory surgery program (and thus not meriting a third party reimbursement rate calculated from the higher costs of providing ambulatory surgical procedures), and the more extensive ambulatory surgery for which specialized resources are necessary.

The plan therefore worked out a system under which hospitals continued to submit claims for covered outpatient surgery visits as before, with the actual procedures described on the routine claim forms. Those hospitals with approved ambulatory rates submit claims for the specific surgical procedures adjudged to be sufficiently major to warrant reimbursement for an ambulatory surgery program; those higher rates are then utilized to reimburse the hospital. For those procedures that do not meet that criterion, the claims are covered by the plan by reimbursing at the hospital's emergency room reimbursement rate.

In the event that a hospital believes that a specific episode warrants the higher rate, despite its not appearing on the plan's list of ambulatory surgical procedures, it is encouraged to submit a medical justification with the claim. If that justification is reasonable, the higher ambulatory surgery rate is paid instead of the lower emergency room rate.

AMBULATORY SURGERY PROCEDURES

Under the system just described, Blue Cross/Blue Shield of Greater New York had to develop a methodology to determine in advance the kinds of procedures that may appropriately be done in an ambulatory surgery program, so as to distinguish them from outpatient procedures that can well be done in hospital clinics and physicians' offices.

The plan, utilizing its own medical staff, conferred with local surgical specialty societies and surgical departments of leading hospitals to develop a *List of Ambulatory Procedures*. Blue Cross/Blue Shield's benefits-administration program uses the list in its computerized claims payment system to sort outpatient surgery claims. Those claims showing procedures on the list are approved for reimbursement at the hospital's ambulatory surgery rate. Claims for surgical procedures not on the list are paid at the emergency room rate.

The initial publication of the list in 1979 elicited a substantial response from hospitals with ambulatory surgery programs and practicing surgeons around the region. Some of the response stemmed from a predictable misunderstanding: Physicians assumed that the plan's purpose was to require the listed procedures to be done on an outpatient basis rather than an inpatient basis. The memorandum accompanying that first publication—and the covering memorandum for each subsequent issuance of revisions of the list plainly states its purpose and points out that the list is specifically meant *not* to be used as a rule of thumb regarding which procedures can be done in which setting.

Much more numerous were the responses from practicing surgeons in particular, who objected either to the inclusion of procedures they believed were appropriate only on an inpatient basis, or to the exclusion of procedures they believed could be done safely and beneficially on an outpatient basis.

Interestingly, although the main purpose of the plan's list was to distinguish between procedures appropriate for a minor clinic or an office and procedures that require an ambulatory surgery program, most of the medical field immediately focused its attention on how to define ambulatory surgery. The main interest was in differentiating between procedures that should only be done on inpatients and those that can sometimes be done appropriately on ambulatory patients.

The result, which has also been affected by evolving medical science, has been periodic revisions of the list. Exhibit 12-1 is the January 1981 publication of the list. For ease of reference, the procedures on the list are grouped under Category I. All other outpatient surgical procedures are under Category II and are reimbursable to the institution at a lower rate of payment.

The generic definition of Category I procedures is:

Ambulatory surgery consists of surgical procedures performed on patients who have not been admitted to hospitals as inpatients. Such procedures require the utilization of a surgical operating room and post-operative recovery room, may require the administration of local or general anesthesia, and must be limited to patients for whom admission as hospital inpatients is not otherwise medically necessary. Ambulatory surgery procedures are limited to those which could appropriately justify admission to a hospital for inpatient services in the absence of an ambulatory surgery program.

Procedures not on the list either are in the Category II level or are of a nature requiring that they ordinarily be performed on an inpatient basis. The list is meant to be used as a guide by each hospital in its application of the ambulatory surgery definition. The plan is in no way advocating that these procedures must be performed on an ambulatory basis; rather it is saying that in most instances, the ambulatory setting may be appropriate and cost-effective.

The list includes some nonsurgical procedures sufficiently complex to warrant their performance in an ambulatory surgery unit. The procedures appear on the list in Exhibit 12–1 in narrative form arranged by classification. The list also exists in alphabetized form with corresponding ICDA–9CM codes.

It should be apparent that although the list has a specific administrative purpose, it also has served a somewhat unexpected additional purpose by stimulating hospital medical staffs to broaden their thinking as to the appropriate uses of ambulatory surgery. Surgeons who write to Blue Cross/ Blue Shield complaining that a particular procedure should not be on the list because it requires two days of postoperative hospitalization may be

Exhibit 12-1 Blue Cross and Blue Shield of Greater New York
List of Ambulatory Procedures

The following list of ambulatory surgery procedures will be reimbursed at the facilities' approved ambulatory surgery rate if done in the ambulatory surgery setting. This list does not constitute a *requirement*; the medical staff of each facility may determine which of these procedures can be done in their ambulatory surgery units.

NERVOUS SYSTEM	Halo type fixation and body cast
	Removal of neroma of cutaneous or digital nerve
	Phrenicotripsy (crushing of phrenic nerves)
	Excision of Morton's neuroma
	Spinal canal injection
	Peripheral nerve suture
	Carpal tunnel release
	Tarsal tunnel release
	Discography
	Biopsy of spine
EYE	Gonio photocoagulation
	Canthotomy—division of canthus, with suture
	Tarsorrhaphy
	Excision major lesion eyelid—full thickness
	Repair of blepharoptosis
	Repair of ectropion or entropion
	Reconstruction of eyelid
	Slitting of lacrimal papilla
	Probing of nasolacrimal duct, with or without irrigation under general anesthesia
	Dacryocystotomy
	Dacryocystotomy—intranasal
	Conjunctivoplasty
	Other free grafts to conjunctiva
	Pterygium removal
	Paracentesis of anterior chamber of eye
	Cyclodialysis
	Discission (needling of lens)
	Aspiration of vitreous
	Repair of retinal detachment with scleral buckling and implant
	Scleral buckling with implant
	Other scleral buckling with air tamponade, resection of sclera, vitrectomy
	Cobalt implant and removal
	Denudation of the cornea for erosion
	Chorioretinal lesion by cryotherapy
	Repair of detached retina
	Cataract extraction
	Excision of xanthelasma
	Excision of herniated fat pad

Exhibit 12-1 continued

EAR	Myringoplasty
	Tympanoplasty
NOSE, MOUTH, PHARYNX	Labial frenotomy
	Excision of dental lesion of jaw
	Suture of laceration of gum
	Excision of lesion or tissue of gum
	Surgical extraction of teeth
	General anesthesia with dental procedures
	Excision of nasal polyps
	Resection of inferior turbinate (submucous)
	Rhinoplasty
	Intranasal antrotomy
	Sinusectomy
	Sialolithotomy (removal of salivary calculus)
	Resection of lip for malignant lesion
	Uvulectomy
	Excision of papilloma, uvula
	Dilation of salivary duct—(ptyalectasis)
	Incision of larynx or trachea
	Thyroglossal duct excision
	Drainage of lingual abscess—other operations on tongue
	Drainage of submaxillary abscess, external approach
	Excision of lesion of maxillary sinus
	Lingual frenotomy
	Lingual frenectomy
	Drainage of face and floor of mouth
	Suture of lacertion of mouth or palate
RESPIRATORY SYSTEM	Excision of tonsil tag(s) (secondary tonsillectomy) with or without adenoidectomy
	Bronchoscopy with therapeutic aspiration of tracheobronchial tree
	Tracheal fenestration with skin flaps
	Laryngoscopy with insertion off radioactive substance
	Bronchoscopy with removal of tumor
	Bronchoscopy with or without biopsy
	Bronchoscopy with removal of foreign body
	Bronchoscopy with injection of contrast medium for bronchography
	Fiberoptic bronchoscopy with or without biopsy
	Closed intrapleural pneumonolysis
	Mediastinoscopy with or without biopsy
	Septoplasty

Exhibit 12-1 continued

RESPIRATORY SYSTEM (cont.)	Adenoidectomy without tonsillectomy Pleural biopsy Tonsillectomy with or without adenoidectomy
CARDIOVASCULAR SYSTEM	Cardiac catheterization Intravenous catheter, by placement in vena cava, right heart or pulmonary artery Ligation of jugular vein, external Ligation of artery and commitant vein or extremity Arterial catheterization for monitoring transfusion or infusion Biopsy of blood vessel (excluding temporal artery) Ligation and stripping of varicose veins Occlusion leg veins Hemodialysis, chronic case Insertion of temporary transvenous electrode Excision of segment of vein of extremity (excluding varicosities)
HEMIC & LYMPHATIC SYSTEMS	Biopsy of lymphatic structure Excision of axillary lymph node Excision of inguinal lymph node Splenic puncture Excision of sternal marrow Excision of deep cervical node or simple excision of chain of lymph nodes
DIGESTIVE SYSTEM	Esophagoscopy with or without biopsy Esophageal biopsy Dilation of esophagus by sound, bougie, bag, indirect, or with pneumatic balloon Gastroscopy with or without biopsy Gastrocamera photo series (as with GE-V) Simple inguinal hernia (Scholdeiss procedure) Unilateral inguinal hernia in infants Flexible fiberoptic colonscopy Large bowel endoscopy Electrocoagulation of villous adenoma transanal approach Closure of other rectal fistula Incision and drainage of supralevator, pulsi-rectal or rectrorectal abscess Incision and drainage of ischiorectal abscess with fistulectomy Destruction of hemorrhoids by cryotherapy Hemorrhoid ligation Closure of anal fistula Sphincterotomy anal—division of anal sphincter

Exhibit 12-1 continued

DIGESTIVE SYSTEM (cont.)	Fistulectomy
	Enucleation or excision of external thrombotic hemorrhoid
	Excision of anal fissure or ulcer
	Aspiration needle biopsy of the liver
	Percutaneous transhepatic cholangiography
	Percutaneous abdominal paracentesis
	Peritoneal dialysis
	Peritoneoscopy with or without biopsy
	Other procedures on hemorrhoids
	Small bowel endoscopy
	Unilateral inguinal hernia
	Fiberoptic esophagoscopy, gastroscopy, and/or esophagoduodenoscopy
	Local excision of lesion or tissue of large intestine
	Colonoscopy
	Excision of colonic polyps
URINARY SYSTEM	Cystoscopy through artificial stoma
	Renal biopsy, percutaneous, by trochar or needle
	Cystourethoscopy with ureteral catheterization
	Excision of urethral caruncle
	Urethral meatomy
MALE GENITAL SYSTEM	Biopsy of prostate, needle or punch, perineal or transrectal approach
	Incisional biopsy of testes
	Excision of local lesion of epididymis
	Excision of varicocele or ligation of spermatic veins for varicocele
	Vasectomy
	Irrigation of corpora cavernosa for priapism
	Circumcision
	Division of penile adhesions
	Excision of spermatocele with or without epididymectomy
FEMALE GENITAL SYSTEM	Dilation of cervical canal
	Biopsy of cervix
	Conization of cervix
	Cryosurgery of cervix
	Tracheloplasty—plastic repair of incompetent cervix (Sherodkar, Baxter or Lash)
	Tracheloplasty—plastic repair of uterine cervix (Emmett)
	Dilatation and Curretage
	Culdocentesis
	Culdotomy

Exhibit 12-1 continued

FEMALE GENITAL SYSTEM (cont.)	Culdoscopy with or without biopsy Excision or other destruction of Bartholin's gland (cyst) Intra-amniotic injection for abortion Bilateral endoscopic occlusion of fallopian tubes Incision or excision of congenital septum of uterus Lysis of intraluminal adhesions of vagina Bilateral fallopian tube destruction Repair of vulvar fistula
MUSCULOSKELETAL SYSTEM	Closed or open reduction of tempromandibular dislocation Other manipulation of tempromandibular joint Closed reduction of fracture with wiring of maxillary teeth Partial ostectomy—metatarsal/tarsal Hammer toe operation Hallux valgus, simple correction by exostectomy (Silver-type procedure) Hallux valgus, radical exostectomy (Keller, McBride or Mays type procedure) Arthrodesis, metatarso-phalangeal joint (bunionette) or interphalangeal joint (toe) Freeing of bone adhesions, callus of synostosis Bone graft, minor or small (e.g., dowell or button), any donor area Arthrotomy (capsulotomy) with exploration, drainage or removal of foreign body Other arthrotomy-elbow Other arthrotomy-knee Other arthrotomy Arthroscopy Shoulder arthroscopy Knee arthroscopy Joint biopsy Incision and drainage of palmar or thenar space Capsulotomy—cutting or division of joint capsule Injection into joint Tenotomy of fingers, major tendon, including cast, minor tendons involving phalanges Suture of quadriceps muscle rupture or biceps muscle rupture Removal of foreign body in muscle Excision of lesion of other soft tissue Excision of tendon sheath Excision of synovial cyst of popliteal space (Baker's cyst)

Exhibit 12-1 continued

MUSCULOSKELETAL SYSTEM (cont.)	Local excision of lesion of muscle (Myositis ossificans, neoplasm)
	Amputation of finger, any joint of phalanx with or without skin graft
	Amputation of metatarsal with toe, or toe at metatarsophalangeal or interphalangeal joint
	Tenosynovectomy of wrist, flexor or extensor tendon sheath
	Partial excision of minor tendons and phalanges
	Foot/toe arthroplasty
	Removal of buried wire, pin, etc.
	Lysis of hand adhesions
	Tenoplasty of hand
	Excision lesion of tendon sheath of hand (ganglionectomy)
	Tenolysis of flexor tendons or fingers
INTEGUMENTARY SYSTEM	Biopsy of breast
	Excision of cyst, fibro-adenoma or other benign tumor, aberrant breast tissue, duct lesion or nipple lesion
	Removal of mammary implant material
	Mastotomy
	Incision pilonidal cyst
	Excision pilonidal cyst
	Debridement of extensive eczematous or infected skin up to 10% of body surface
	Removal of malignant lesion by any method, except radiotherapy or chemotherapy
	Excision and/or repair by Z-plasty
	Excision and/or repair by rotation flap, advanced flap, double, pedicle flap, etc.
	Primary attachment of open or tubed pedicle flap to recipient site requiring minimal preparation
	Intermediate delay of any flap, primary delay, small flap or sectioning pedicle of tubed direct flap
	Pinch split, or full thickness skin graft to cover small ulcer, tip or digit up to defect size ¾ inch (1.8 cm) diameter
	Split skin graft, trunk, scalp, arms, legs, hands and feet up to 12 sq. inches
	Destruction of large lesion
	Incision with exploration or drainage of deep abscess
	Excision of lipoma
	Argon laser for destruction of congenital hemangioma

Exhibit 12-1 continued

| DIAGNOSTIC & THERAPEUTIC PROCEDURES | Myelogram
Angiocardiography
Intra-arterial injection, carotid or vertebral
Arteriography
Insertion or removal of wire or pin for skeletal traction
Application of calipers or tongs
Implant of P32
Implant and removal of cobalt
Esophagoscopy with foreign body removal
Gastroscopy with foreign body removal
Arteriogram: retrograde, brachial, aortic or femoral
Indirect laryngoscopy with removal of foreign body
Examination of eyes of infant under general anesthesia
Transfusion of blood and blood components
Plasmopheresis
Cytopheresis
Percutaneous hepatic cholangiogram
Electroshock therapy
Laparoscopy |

Source: Blue Cross and Blue Shield of Greater New York, January 1981

informed by the plan that a half-dozen prestigious hospitals in the region routinely perform the procedure on an outpatient basis. This fact often can stimulate a change in patterns of practice.

UTILIZATION REVIEW AND QUALITY ASSURANCE

It is the basic policy of Blue Cross/Blue Shield of Greater New York that the responsibilities for reviewing the utilization of hospital services and for assuring the quality of medical services lie primarily with each hospital or other health care facility. This policy applies as much to ambulatory surgery as to inpatient services, and to freestanding, independent facilities as well as to hospitals. Typically, each facility delegates this responsibility to its own medical staff's peer review structures, with appropriate administrative and technical support.

The plan expects that each hospital's utilization review and medical care evaluation programs will review the appropriateness and quality of ambulatory surgery on an ongoing basis. In addition, Blue Cross/Blue Shield conducts a retrospective review of ambulatory surgery utilization. That review yields two important by-products: hospital profiles, and further revisions that need to be made to the list. The plan shares their utilization data with the hospitals.

Without the professional integrity of a vigorous peer review program, there is little assurance that an ambulatory surgery program will contribute positively to the community's health, and there is no assurance that the program will not add to costs rather than show savings.

An insufficiently noted development of the past decade is the increasing rigor the JCAH has demanded of institutions granting surgical privileges to members of their medical staffs. It is no longer common for the appointments of surgical specialists to be delineated simply as "full privileges," wherein there is implicit reliance on informal peer pressures in the surgical suite and on the individual surgeon's own professional integrity to assure that there will be no attempt to perform procedures in which substantial proficiency has not been demonstrated.

Hospitals almost universally extend the discipline of their inpatient surgical service to the ambulatory surgery program as well. It is clearly absurd to permit surgeons to perform procedures on outpatients that would be proscribed or limited if they were to be performed on inpatients. For this reason Blue Cross/Blue Shield of Greater New York, in its *Guidelines for Freestanding Ambulatory Surgery Facilities,* insists that nonhospital units "have a formally organized medical staff functioning under rules and regulations . . . including procedures for delineating the scope of professional practice permitted for each member of the medical staff. . . . [Members] should each have appointments with equivalent delineated privileges at one or more hospitals in the area.[3(pXX)]

The plan's insistence on these safeguards, as well as on a rigorous utilization review, is based on a simple premise. The increased safety and the cost-savings of ambulatory surgery would be wiped out if freestanding, independent facilities become a haven for surgeons to perform procedures that would be limited or prohibited at local hospitals because of utilization standards or practice limitations.

If a local hospital, for example, at the insistence of its pediatric service, establishes strict clinical criteria for the performance of tonsillectomies and adenoidectomies, that important quality assurance measure would be essentially negated if one or more otorhinolaryngologists (or nonspecialist surgeons) shifted these procedures to a nearby freestanding facility. Similarly, if a hospital's surgical department places restrictions on the performance of certain complex procedures, that effort would be largely in vain if surgeons continued to carry out those procedures unsupervised at a separate nonhospital facility. It is of interest that the federal government's new ambulatory surgery policy, with respect to Medicare beneficiaries (as described in Chapter 1), now embodies the principles of linking the practice in freestanding, independent facilities of authorizing the performance of the same procedure in a nearby hospital to the requirement of a utilization review.

In the seventeen-county service area of Blue Cross/Blue Shield of Greater New York, a half-dozen freestanding, independent facilities have become participating ambulatory surgical units under contract with the plan. All the facilities are specialized, limiting their services to such procedures as pregnancy terminations, vasectomies, and so on. No comprehensive facilities of the surgery center variety have developed in the region; discussions occur from time to time with proprietary facilities that are used by surgeons in fields such as cosmetic surgery and otology, but to date, none have sought participating status with the plan.

COST SAVINGS

An extended research effort is under way through the plan's Health Affairs Research Department to establish the dollar-savings involved in the ambulatory surgery initiative. This effort is considerably more complex than merely comparing the dollars paid to the facilities for ambulatory surgical procedures with the dollars that would have been paid if the same procedures had been done on an inpatient basis. That comparison does show substantial savings in benefits payments. For the findings to be truly meaningful, however, data on the actual costs incurred by the institutions must be studied, as must the utilization patterns and the ripple effects of these changes on reimbursement rates.

It is not intended that this effort be aimed at the publication of an elegant research monograph. Rather, the activity is meant to provide the plan with useful management information for mapping out its practices in administering the benefit, and for planning its continuing efforts to encourage all hospitals to develop ambulatory surgery programs. In time, however, research papers will be published.

REFERENCES

1. Blue Cross/Blue Shield of Greater New York: *Guidelines for Freestanding Ambulatory Care Facilities*. New York, Blue Cross/Blue Shield of Greater New York, 1977.
2. Blue Cross Association: *Relationships between Blue Cross Plans and Freestanding Ambulatory Care Facilities*. New York, Blue Cross Association, Oct. 27, 1972; revised and reissued as *Revised Statement of Policy Regarding Relationships between Blue Cross Plans and*

Freestanding Ambulatory Care Facilities. Blue Cross/Blue Shield Association, New York, 1981.

3. Blue Cross/Blue Shield of Greater New York: *Guidelines for Freestanding Ambulatory Surgery Facilities*. New York, Blue Cross/Blue Shield of Greater New York, 1981.

4. Joint Commission on Accreditation of Hospitals: *Accreditation Manual for Hospitals, 1982 Edition*. Chicago, Joint Commission on Accreditation of Hospitals, 1979.

Chapter 13

Designing Financial Incentives for Ambulatory Surgery

Mark V. Pauly, Ph.D. and
Linda A. Burns, M.H.A.

Often surgery can be performed either in an inpatient or an outpatient (ambulatory) setting. Using an ambulatory setting may affect the cost associated with performing a given surgical procedure. In addition, the availability of ambulatory settings may affect the total cost for surgeries by affecting the total number of surgeries performed. This chapter discusses two topics related to these observations. First, the discussion focuses on what is known and what could be known about the costs of certain surgical procedures performed in an inpatient as compared with an outpatient setting. Second, the discussion outlines the kinds of financial incentives to patients and physicians that would induce the former to use an ambulatory program and the latter to perform surgery in the most appropriate setting and to carry out the optimum total number of surgeries in each setting. An analysis will be made of the impact of financial incentives on the setting in which surgery is performed and on the total number of surgeries performed.

Although relatively little is known empirically about these issues, it will be helpful to summarize what is known. The primary objective of this chapter, therefore, is to pose questions rather than to answer them. Posing proper questions in the proper way, however, is the first step toward obtaining correct answers. In fact, claims sometimes made for supporting particular financing arrangements require that specific questions be answered before the financing arrangements are implemented.

FACTS AND FALLACIES ABOUT AMBULATORY SURGERY

Of the 19.9 million surgical procedures performed in U.S. short-term general hospitals, 18 percent were performed in ambulatory settings in 1981.[1] There also is an unknown amount of ambulatory surgery performed in nonhospital settings, such as freestanding, independent surgical centers and independent private physician's offices. Recently released data revealed that 552,895 ambulatory surgical procedures were performed in freestanding, independent ambulatory surgical centers in 1981.[2] Within undefined limits of safety or acceptability, industry observers have speculated that 20 to 40 percent of all surgical procedures in the United States could be performed in an ambulatory setting.[3]

What impact would such a change have on the cost of medical care in the United States? That costs would be less is the apparently obvious answer. After all, unlike inpatient surgery, ambulatory surgery does not require the use of a hospital's inpatient accommodations. With charges for an inpatient stay averaging $325 per day,[4] the avoidance of even one day of stay for each surgical case transferred to an outpatient setting would save 2.5 billion dollars in hospital charges per year. Altering reimbursement and payment incentives to encourage ambulatory surgery therefore would seem to be an easy conclusion. Paying surgeons relatively more for ambulatory surgery and/or making it relatively less costly than inpatient surgery to patients would seem to be obvious solutions.

There are reasons, however, that these conclusions may not be foregone; the design of appropriate incentives may be *more* complex than is immediately apparent. The dilemma is that public policy makers want to encourage surgery in an ambulatory setting only when it is lower in cost and is properly performed. The simple financial incentives mentioned above are blunt and dull instruments; they often cannot be used to make as fine a distinction as we would like between appropriate and inappropriate surgical cases.

The fundamental problem is that in establishing a reimbursement and payment system, policy makers are limited to making the reimbursement level dependent on the objectively observable and verifiable characteristics of a situation. (Indeed, there may even be some cost in observing or verifying these characteristics.) It is unlikely that ambulatory surgery will be the preferred choice in all situations having a particular set of characteristics. Ambulatory surgery may be most appropriate some of the time, most of the time, or almost all of the time; but there will be special cases in which ambulatory surgery will not be appropriate. In these cases, surgery should be performed either in an inpatient setting or not at all. Financial incentives, however, would reward ambulatory surgery whether a case is ordinary or special. Policy makers may be willing to make a trade off by exchanging a few inappropriate decisions for a much larger number of appropriate ones. One could argue that even if medical care would not be perfect under a new set of incentives, society would at least be better off than it is now under present incentives. Nevertheless, in any practical setting, the critical point is that using financial incentives to affect medical practice requires care. Some harm, along with the good, will surely arise.

Ideal reimbursement and payment policies for ambulatory surgery, then, require discovering two kinds of information. First, policy makers must determine the circumstances in which ambulatory surgery is almost always or usually as good as or better than inpatient surgery or alternative forms of therapy. Then, a method must be chosen for paying patients and physicians so as to encourage use of an ambulatory setting. The more certain policy makers can be about the appropriateness of the setting, the less careful one needs to be about the specific design of the financial incentives. The following sections review what is known and needs to be known about two issues—the appropriateness of ambulatory surgery and the design of financial incentives.

Although there is no question that a sizable number of surgeries— probably more than at present—could be performed in an ambulatory setting without obvious reduction in patient safety, policy makers must be cautious in concluding that it is therefore preferable to do so. Two additional and related questions must be asked to guard against some fallacies or mistakes. First, are the resource costs of ambulatory surgery less than those of the alternative form of therapy, and, if so, by how much? Second, does the patient prefer the alternative to ambulatory surgery, and, if so, how much is the patient willing to pay for the alternative? More than "medical equivalence" is required; one must also consider the amenities (plus or minus) that accrue to patients from alternative forms of therapy. In each case, of course, it is assumed that a patient is properly informed. Some examples will illustrate the kinds of fallacies that can occur.

Fallacy 1: Explicit Charges Measure All Costs

Suppose that the only acceptable alternative to ambulatory surgery is inpatient surgery. The question then is, What are the total costs of the resources consumed in each of these two settings? Some of the costs are presumably the same, since the same actions in the surgical suite and recovery room are performed. Other actions are different, and the costs are therefore different. The inpatient surgical patient, for example, may spend a preoperative night in the hospital, and may convalesce as an inpatient for some days after the surgery. The basic question is, What differences in real resource use exist between the two forms of surgery? It is important to realize that these differences often are *not* reflected in differences in charges billed and paid. Consider, for example, the period of convalescence following inpatient surgery in uncomplicated cases. The patients may be charged the same hospital room-and-board rate that all inpatients are charged, but if their surgery was not complex and if they recover rapidly, they probably *consume* less than the average amount of resources per day, such as nursing time. Then the actual marginal cost of their inpatient convalescence is the cost of the additional personnel time of registered nurses, nurse aides, and other ancillary personnel the patients' presence requires, plus the cost of meals, administration, and drugs, supplies, and dressings. In contrast, if the patients convalesced outside the hospital (e.g., at home), there would be an implicit cost associated with having family members care for the patients, or the explicit cost of a private duty nurse or aide hired for this purpose. There would be the implict cost of preparing meals and, possibly, of bedroom "rental." This "rent" is dependent on the availability of needed space. The implicit costs represent the value that the provider of a "free" input would have placed on the input in its next best use. If a family member had to stay home from work and assist the patient, for example, the cost would be the family member's lost wages. Even if the family member sacrificed only leisure or household time, it would surely be time worth something.

To the extent that candidates for ambulatory surgery use fewer hospital nursing inputs per day than the average patient, and to the extent that they consume inputs at home, where costs are implicit rather than explicit, the difference in charges between the two settings may overstate greatly the differences in real costs. There may be little if any cost-saving, especially if the hospital does not reduce staffing much in the event that patients use an ambulatory setting instead of an inpatient setting.

These possibilities should not be overemphasized, however; certainly there are real and substantial cost-savings to be gained from ambulatory surgery. Policy makers must nonetheless be careful in drawing conclusions based on a comparison of charges, precisely because charges do not necessarily equal real marginal costs. The strongest argument for substitution of ambulatory surgery for inpatient surgery would be a surgical case in which the ambulatory surgery candidate actually would receive, as an inpatient, services that consumed real resources, such as tests and nursing services, even though the services provided the patient with no benefit; that is the services were performed, perhaps, only as a matter of routine hospital and medical practice. Then these services would represent resources used in a wasteful way, and this waste could be eliminated by ambulatory surgery.

Fallacy 2: Only Medical Appropriateness Is Relevant

The second aspect that needs comparison between inpatient and outpatient settings is patient benefits including patient amenities. Patients, for example, who would prefer not to impose on their families during a period of convalescence would not be suitable for ambulatory surgery and recovery at home. The preference for amenities, of course, can be for those at either setting; the main point is that patient preferences need to be taken into account. Different forms of treatment would be appropriate for people with identical medical conditions but with different preferences.

Fallacy 3: The Tyranny of the Typical

This final point is often overlooked. In determining which type of treatment is appropriate, policy makers should examine unusual as well as usual cases. Suppose, for example, that in 99 percent of all surgeries of a given type, uncomplicated cases can convalesce without problems equally well as outpatients or inpatients. Suppose further that patients prefer to be at home and that care there is less costly in real terms. In addition, suppose complications do occur in 1 percent of the cases, and that the patient who is not in the hospital convalescing must be rushed by ambulance to the emergency department, at additional cost and with additional psychological stress and pain. The choice of proper setting obviously requires taking this possibility into account by comparing expected or average costs (of all 100 cases), and by considering how the patient feels about the minimal chance of having to be transported by ambulance to the hospital emergency department.

All these aspects of care need to be taken into account before deciding whether or not it would be better to encourage ambulatory surgery. Because people differ in terms of their preference for amenities, their implicit costs, and whether or not they will become the unusual complicated case, it is quite likely that not all persons with the same objective characteristics can be best cared for in one setting over another. What we do not know is whether there are circumstances in which many people now receive inpatient surgery but for which almost all would be better off with ambulatory surgery. There may be many cases in which the patients would be no worse off—or only a little worse off—in terms of amenities, but their cost saving would more than compensate. These are the cases for which ambulatory surgery should be encouraged, although it is recognized that, whichever setting is encouraged, there are bound to be some mistakes.

ENCOURAGING AMBULATORY SURGERY: HOW AND TO WHOM

If ambulatory surgery is nearly as good as inpatient surgery but has a much lower real cost, why should it need to be encouraged? To answer this question, it is necessary to look at current incentives for patients and providers.

Incentives for Patients

The primary reason, at least in theory, as to why surgery may not be performed in the proper setting is because of defective incentives to patients. The reason is simple: Patients who elect the lowest (real) cost setting do not usually obtain the benefit from that lower cost. Health insurance commonly covers the cost of surgery in full, regardless of the setting, but often does not cover the implicit cost or the cost of convalescence at home. Sometimes health insurance even pays less of the physicians's fee. From the patient's viewpoint, ambulatory surgery is not obviously better than inpatient surgery, and it often costs even more either in explicit, out-of-pocket costs or in implicit costs. Current reimbursement and payment policies fail to let patients share in the cost-saving advantages of ambulatory surgery. To be sure, if there are cost-savings, premiums would fall if more surgery is done on an ambulatory basis. But the premium of an individual who is insured does not fall perceptibly if ambulatory surgery is elected. Consequently, patients should not be expected to choose ambulatory surgery, even when it is to their advantage to do so. The first type of alteration in incentives, therefore, should concentrate on incentives to patients.

Incentives to Surgeons

The predominant practice is to pay the surgeon the same amount regardless of where the patient receives preoperative and postoperative care. Some insurance companies actually pay less if the patient is not an inpatient, especially if the surgery itself occurs in a setting outside a hospital, such as a freestanding, independent surgical center or a physician's office. Some insurance companies do pay a modest additional amount for ambulatory surgery, designated as a facility fee.

The net return to the surgeon depends on more than the gross revenue received; it also depends on the surgeon's costs. For surgery performed in an outpatient setting independent of a hospital, there may be explicit costs associated with the surgery itself (assistants, supplies, space) for which the surgeon must pay but for which cost-based reimbursement is typically not available. In addition, it may take more of the physician's time to care for the ambulatory surgery patient, who is not conveniently available in the hospital for daily rounds, than to care for the inpatient surgical patient.

These observations suggest that there is usually no increase, and there may be a decrease, in net income per surgical procedure for the surgeon who uses the outpatient setting. It could be argued that this situation makes little difference, since surgeons do what is best for their patients and act (in economic terminology) as the patients' true agent. First, in many cases there is little or no medical difference between surgical settings. Excluding the possibility of hospital-borne infections, the hospital inpatient setting is rarely a worse setting. As noted above, when the patient gains financially from using the hospital inpatient surgery, it may be better for both patient and surgeon even though it is worse for society. Second, there are likely to be cases—ones that are medically ambiguous or in which physicians are in financial distress—when financial considerations do matter and take precedence, at the margin, over small improvements in patient comfort or outcome.

Incentives to the Hospital

Surgery can be performed in the hospital's surgical suites, with convalescence occurring either in the hospital for inpatients or outside for outpatients, since most hospitals have the capability to provide both inpatient and ambulatory surgery. Obviously, the hospital will generate more total revenue if it can retain the patient for an inpatient stay. In addition, if the insurance company pays charges, and if hospital charges exceed its marginal cost for days of stay, the hospital may generate profits from an inpatient stay. If the choice is between surgery on an inpatient basis or on an ambulatory basis, current insurance arrangements obviously permit the hospital to gain more if surgery occurs on an inpatient rather than on an outpatient basis.

Even if the hospital in some sense gains from inpatient surgery and inpatient stays, however, it is unclear how this gain can be translated into actions or advice that affect the patient. There is likely to be some link between what is good for the hospital and what the attending physician or surgeon wants to do, though the connection is not likely to be very direct. It is true, however, that under current reimbursement policies, the hospital surely does not have an incentive to discourage inpatient surgery admissions and length-of-stays.

Incentives for Other Physicians

Most, though by no means all, surgery patients are initially recommended to surgeons or referred by another physician—often an internist, pediatrician, or general or family practitioner. Present payment and reimbursement policies provide little incentive for these primary care physicians to favor ambulatory surgery over inpatient surgery. It is possible that the nonhospital patient may be more likely to use the nonsurgeon's services than the inpatient still under the surgeon's care; but, on the other hand, the referring physician may also have a preference for the convenience of in-hospital rounds and consultations. Finally, to the extent that ambulatory surgery may cost their patients money and inconvenience, referring physcians may bear the brunt (and perhaps even the consequences) of patient complaints.

Incentives To Perform Surgery or Not

The discussion to this point has considered only the possibility of substituting outpatient surgery for inpatient surgery, and the cost-savings that accrue. In many cases, such a substitution is attractive; but often the surgical setting is not the only choice to be made. There may be, for example, a nonsurgical form of treatment that is even more economical and as good as, or only a little worse than, ambulatory surgery. The dilemma is that financial incentives (to the patient or the physician) intended to encourage ambulatory surgery as a substitute for inpatient surgery may also encourage more surgery in total. In economic terminology, it would be necessary to look at the "own-price" effect as well as at the "cross-price" effect.

There are some indications that policy makers need to be cautious in this regard. The same kinds of arguments about encouraging the substitution of more economical forms of care have been used to justify expanding insurance coverage for extended-care facilities or for doctor office visits. In virtually every case, the own-price effect was so large that total costs increased, despite the fact that there was some substitution.

The same situation could occur with ambulatory surgery. This occurence would be especially likely in areas where there is presently an excess demand on hospital beds or surgical suites. Providing better coverage for ambulatory care, or coverage for surgery done on an outpatient basis, is a way of lifting the resource constraint (which a health systems agency with certificate-of-need requirements may have consciously selected). The likely rise in costs is necessarily a negative outcome but is one that should be anticipated.

Designing Incentives

There are many ways in which ambulatory surgery in different settings can be made more attractive relative to inpatient surgery. From an economic perspective, the choice with regard to substitution depends primarily on the relative price for care at each type of location. A second issue is whether incentives are to be offered to patients, to providers (hospitals and physicians), or to both. The third issue is whether the incentive is to be selective—that is, applicable only to situations with certain characteristics—or more generalized.

It may be useful to distinguish three kinds of potential surgical situations: those for which outpatient surgery is very rarely appropriate; those for which outpatient surgery is almost always appropriate or acceptable; and those in which outpatient surgery may be appropriate or inappropriate.

The first category—very complex surgeries where the patient requires a great deal of follow up—obviously requires no alterations in current incentives. The second category is more interesting, although there may be more arguments about which actual cases fit into this group. One can then catalog incentives as to whether they affect patient or provider, and whether they involve an increase in present coverage for ambulatory surgery or a reduction in coverage for inpatient surgery. Table 13-1 shows most of the possibilities in matrix form.

Cell 1 considers increasing the user price by reducing the insurance coverage for inpatient surgery. This adjustment could result in higher out-of-pocket payments by the patient for both the surgeon's fees and the hospital's charge. Because the hospital's charge for an inpatient stay usually greatly exceeds all professional fees, raising the level of copayment for inpatient hospital care for those procedures in which ambulatory surgery is likely to be appropriate may be the most effective incentive for the patient.

Cell 2 could involve such strategies as having an insurance with a higher "reasonable and customary charge"maximum for having surgery performed on an outpatient basis; for having low or zero copayments (but positive copayments for inpatient therapy); or for having the insurance

---

Table 13-1 Classification of Incentives for Ambulatory Surgery

Incentives	Reducing Insurance Coverage of Inpatient Surgery	Increasing Insurance Coverage of Ambulatory Surgery
Patients	1	2
Surgeons	3	4
Hospitals	5	6

Source: Mark V. Pauly and Linda A. Burns.

cover part of the expense for convalescence at home, such as home health visits and housekeeper services. An even simpler approach would simply be to make a cash payment bonus to the patient who elects ambulatory rather than inpatient surgery. Given the discomfort and risk of many types of surgery, and given the real cost of convalescence, it is unlikely that a modest "reward" would encourage an increase in the total number of surgeries; but it could have an important impact on the setting where surgery is performed. In effect, the bonus is a kind of incentive reimbursement arrangement in which the benefits from cost-savings are shared with patients. The financial attractiveness of such a scheme is critically dependent on how responsive patients would be to financial incentives as to the choice of place of surgery.

Usually there is some link between the insurance coverage that patients receive and the generosity of reimbursement and payments to providers, though it is possible to separate these influences somewhat. For surgeons, reductions in either the level of insurance reimbursement or the maximum fee they are permitted to collect could discourage inpatient surgery. Reduction in the level of reimbursement would have the advantage of combining surgeon and patient incentives that point in the same direction. In contrast, retaining levels of patient payment at, say, zero dollars out-of-pocket but reducing what the surgeon can receive for inpatient surgery is more likely to set up a conflict of incentives, since the patient will still have no financial deterrent to inpatient surgery. Thus cell 3 may be best filled by setting the surgeon's payment at a lower rate for inpatient surgery than for the same surgery performed on an ambulatory basis. Where surgeons are currently paid less if a procedure is done on an ambulatory basis, a strategy in cell 4 would involve paying at least as much, according to established surgical fee schedules. It may even be appropriate to pay somewhat more for the procedure done on an ambulatory basis in order to reflect the possibly higher real costs of such surgery. When the surgery is performed in a freestanding, independent surgical center, an additional amount could also be added as coverage of the nonsurgeon costs included in the surgeon's fee.

Cells 5 and 6 would involve adjusting hospital reimbursement to pay less than costs or charges for inpatient surgery, and to be especially generous (perhaps even pay a "profit") toward hospital charges incurred through ambulatory surgery. The desirability of such courses of action depends on what one assumes about the ability of hospitals to influence the amount of outpatient surgery; there is a danger of punishing or rewarding hospitals financially for decisions that are primarily made by physicians. The case for rewards and penalties is strongest for those hospitals that could set up ambulatory surgery programs or facilities but have not yet done so, or that have adopted general rules or are managed in a way that discourages ambulatory surgery.

These incentives would be most appropriate for those types of surgical procedures for which ambulatory surgery is likely to be most appropriate. There will be a set of "in-between" or "gray-area" procedures where such surgery is sometimes appropriate and sometimes not. The incentives just described could, in such judgmental cases, turn patient or physician choices away from what is most beneficial in terms of costs and benefits.

There are several ways to sharpen the effectiveness of financial incentives. For patients, one possibility would be to have a uniform nonzero copayment for inpatient and outpatient surgery set at a level that the patient could still afford to pay (probably varying with income). Paying 20 percent of the hospital bill, for example, where the hospital bill for inpatient surgery is four times greater than for outpatient surgery, would lead to a level of out-of-pocket payment that is four times higher than if the patient selects outpatient surgery. Such a copayment may also help to encourage less expensive nonsurgical forms of therapy as well.

For surgeons, the objective probably should be to try to achieve financial neutrality; that is, reimbursement should be structured so that the surgeon receives about the same net income regardless of where the surgery is performed. (This situation differs from the cases discussed earlier, where the objective was to yield the surgeon a higher net income under the ambulatory surgery strategy.) The presumption, therefore, is that the surgeon's interest in the patient's welfare will wholly determine the choice; the surgeon will not have financial incentives to compromise the patient's best interests. Perfect neutrality is not going to be possible, of course, but adjusting surgeon reimbursements to be proportionate to the average total implicit cost for each procedure is probably worthwhile.

Adjusting the financial incentives for inpatient versus ambulatory surgery is not going to have a large effect on the total number of surgeries performed, regardless of the location, unless those adjustments appreciably affect the average (of all locations) level of copayment paid or the average level of fee or reimbursement received. When an insurer can take account of the total cost of care, as in a health maintenance organization, there can be financial incentives to do less surgery more economically. This incentive can be too strong, of course. In any case, the desired adjustment in overall fee or reimbursement levels depends on the insurer's judgment regarding the appropriateness of current surgery rates, regardless of the surgery setting.

How Can Change Be Achieved?

Suppose the conclusion is reached—based on the incomplete available data and on intuition—that more ambulatory surgery would be a good idea. It would save more in costs than it would reduce patient welfare, if it would reduce welfare at all. It may also be concluded that the new financial incentives outlined in the previous sections would be a good way to encourage more ambulatory surgery. It would be easy to assert that policy makers should enact a series of regulations on insurance benefit packages that, in effect, would require insurers to do what is right. Insurers, for example, could be forbidden from paying less to the surgeon for ambulatory surgery, and copayments could be required for inpatient surgery.

A preferable strategy, however, may be one that is more indirect. If ambulatory surgery and the financial incentives that may encourage it really are better, the world should not require regulations to encourage it to beat a path to the door of innovation. The competitive market test should be sufficient to obtain the proper rate of diffusion. If the new reimbursement structures suggested in this chapter would be effective, then competitive insurers should be eager to adopt them, since they would permit the insurer to offer a more attractive benefit package at a lower premium. From this perspective, the chapter discussion would be viewed as an encouragement and not a prescription.

There are, of course, some responses and objections to this naive market-test rule. One response is to note that ambulatory surgery is already diffusing at a rapid rate, so that the speculation here is more in the nature of forecasting how insurance coverage could be expected to respond. Another objection is that current forms of insurance coverage may not be competitively determined. If ambulatory surgery really does cut costs, it reduces total revenues run through the medical care sector. Neither hospitals nor physicians collectively would be especially enthusiastic about such a prospect. The dominance of the insurance market in many states by provider-controlled Blue Cross/Blue Shield plans and the alleged influence that providers exert on commercial businesses may be sufficient to discourage the emergence of a (competitively) better method for financing surgical procedures. The problem with this objection is that we do not know whether it is legitimate. Even if it is, the remedy is not to regulate benefit packages but to remove monopoly power, which is illegal in any case.

A third response is that ambulatory surgery really is better, but people—insurers, health professionals, and consumers—need to be made aware of it. If this assertion is true, the process of diffusion would only be a matter of time. One useful public activity, however, would be to support investigations of the effectiveness of financial incentives. The types of conditions for which ambulatory surgery does lower real costs, not just charges, and the distribution of patients, within any diagnosis category, who would be made better or worse off, and by how much, are all things that need to be known. In addition, a crucial point related to one earlier discussion is how responsive providers and consumers will be to financial incentives. If an insurer offers a bonus for ambulatory surgery but the bonus is primarily claimed by those who would have had ambulatory surgery anyway, such an incentive scheme will be much less attractive than if the bonus motivated a great deal of substitution. Virtually nothing is known about the magnitude of changes in behavior that benefit packages or reimbursement changes would create. This information is something that few private insurers would find worthwhile to generate on their own, and yet it is essential to the appropriate design of insurance plans.

Ambulatory Surgery and the Competitive Health Care System

A final reason why sufficient ambulatory surgery, and the insurance that encourages it, may not yet exist is related to the current arguments for more competitive arrangements in health insurance. Suppose new incentives for ambulatory surgery would trim forty dollars a month off an employee's health insurance premium. If the employer were paying the premium but the labor market was competitive, one could expect most of the forty dollars eventually to show up in the employee's cash wages. But there is an important difference: the forty dollars in cash would be subject to income and payroll taxes, whereas the forty dollars in health insurance premiums would be untaxed. If ambulatory surgery is regarded as less attractive on the average in terms of amenities, or if there is inertia, the fact that some of the cost-savings will disappear in taxes may be sufficient to discourage the adoption of the better benefit package.

Employees, moreover, would be less likely to choose such an option on their own if the employer paid the full premium for whatever benefit package was selected. In contrast, if the employer made a fixed-dollar contribution, individual employees might place higher value on the option of choosing benefits that encourage ambulatory surgery.

The competition approach to containing health care expenditures involves removal of tax deductibility, at least for changes in benefit packages, and possibly requiring or encouraging fixed-dollar employer contributions. Such changes could be expected to enhance the attractiveness to employers and employees of such cost-cutting devices as ambulatory surgery, whether or not those devices are encouraged by changes in the fee-for-service benefit package or embodied in the protocols chosen by cost-conscious health maintenance organizations.

Providers and insurers who want to anticipate appropriate responses in such a competitive system would be well advised to consider ambulatory surgery and benefits that encourage it. Although more remains to be known about the magnitude of these benefits, there is sufficient promise to justify considerable interest.

REFERENCES

1. American Hospital Association: *Hospital Statistics, 1982 Edition.* Chicago, American Hospital Association, 1982, p 8.

2. Statistics presentation at the Eighth Annual Meeting of the Freestanding Ambulatory Surgical Association. April 1, 1982, Washington, DC, Freestanding Ambulatory Surgical Association, April 1, 1982.

3. Davis JE, Detmer DE: The ambulatory surgery unit. *Ann Surg* 1972; 175:856.

4. American Hospital Association: National panel survey, (unpublished). Chicago, American Hospital Association, 1982.

Index

E

Emergency department: relationship of ambulatory surgery to, 97-98; site for ambulatory surgery program, 121; use of waiting area for ambulatory surgery patient's family, 101; benefits, 177; mentioned, 180

Emergency room. *See* emergency department

Endoscopy: ambulatory procedures, 55

F

Facility architectural program details functional space requirements, 113

Facility case study A: a freestanding, hospital affiliated unit, 88-96

Facility case study B: hospital owned and integrated into hospital, 97

Facility charge: *See* facility fee

Facility fee: defined, 15; posted, 156; mentioned, 45

Facility planning: success requires knowledge of planning, design and construction, 107

Facility type: hospital programs, 7-8; freestanding, 120-121; integrated with hospital, 120-121

Facility: benefits from location on campus, 49

Facility: codes, 110-111; regulations, 108

Facility: conformity with codes necessary for reimbursement, 179

Facility: construction administration, 119; contract documents, 119; construction, new, 119-120; renovated, 119-120

Facility: cost comparisons using value engineering, 110

Facility: description of ambulatory surgery space requirements, 109; functional analysis, 116; space relationships, 115-116

Facility: design lessons learned, 104-105; criteria for selection of options, 85; criteria for design, 86; concepts, 122-125

Facility: design options/models defined, 83; freestanding independent, 83; freestanding facility, 83; freestanding facility connected to a hospital, 83; facility integrated into hospital, 83

Facility: financial feasibility of, 112

Facility: flow patterns, 114

Facility: project delivery, 112

Facility: size, 97

Facility: staff areas features, 92

Family role: discharge of patient, 168; responsibility for patient, 173

Ferber, M.S.: mentioned, 49

Financial incentives: purpose of, 195; design of, 202-205; for patients, 200; for surgeons, 200-201; to hospitals, 201; to physicians, 201-202; to perform or not to perform surgery, 202; trade-offs, 196; need for research in, 206-207

Financial statements: Crouse-Irving Memorial Hospital, 147-148

Financing: shifts in site of surgical care, 45; *See* reimbursement

Focus group: role of, 31-32

Ford, J.: mentioned, 11, 35, 43

Freestanding Ambulatory Surgical Association: data from, 11-12; accreditation, 162; mentioned, 44

Freestanding ambulatory surgery centers: defined, 3

Freestanding, independent surgery centers: justification for, 153; efficiency, 49; birthing centers, 177

G

General surgery: ambulatory
procedures, 53
Geographic location: hospital
programs, 7
Georgetown University Hospital:
mentioned, 168, 169, 170
Gonella, J.: mentioned, 75
Governance: involvement in planning,
37
Graduate Medical Education National
Advisory Committee: physician
manpower, 60
Group Health Association of
America, Inc.: accreditation, 162
Gynecology: data on use, 51

H

Health Insurance Association of
America: policy toward ambulatory
surgery, 16-17; recommends
coverage, 156
Health System Agency: hearings,
158, 160; law reviewed, 14;
mentioned, 22
Hersfeld, G.: mentioned, 35
Hertzler: mentioned, 49
Hess, L.: mentioned, 171
Hill, C.: mentioned, 10, 43
Hospital control defined: hospital
sponsored, 3: hospital associated,
3; hospital as landlord, 3; high
degree, 2; low degree, 2
Hospital involvement: reasons for, 4;
capabilities for ambulatory surgery,
127-128
House officers: participation in
ambulatory surgery, 58

I

Image: of facility, 116
In-and-out surgery. *See* ambulatory
surgery
Ingall, J.R.F.: mentioned, 160
Inpatient operating rooms: use for
ambulatory surgery, 101
Insurance: benefits tax deductible,
207; coverage from patient's
perspective, 168; coverage for
ambulatory surgery, 131-132; mix
of payers, 149

J

Joint Commission on Accreditation of
Hospitals: innovation encouraged
in solving problems in quality
assurance, 65; standing orders, 40;
quality assurance, 64;
recommendations for quality
assurance program, 68; written
standards of care, 77; standards
reviewed, 12-13; mentioned, 110,
172, 180

K

Kansas Blue Cross: benefits, 156
Knauer, Virginia: mentioned, 22

L

Lang, Norma: mentioned, 64-65
Legal issues: malpractice, 51;
summary, 14-15
Licensure: reviewed, 14
Location defined: hospital based, 3;
satellite, 3
Long-range plan: Presbyterian
Hospital of Dallas, 135